"Most of us have wrestled with a loved one's death by cancer, and when surprised by life, celebrate it. But Alec Hill takes us deeper. Diving beneath the surface of the good news of survival, he exposes the emotions and challenges when side-stepping death. And from his own journey and those of others, Alec teaches the cancer survivor how to thrive in the unexpected gift of bonus years. This, however, is not just a book for those surviving a life-threatening disease; Alec teaches us all how to live."

Sharol Hayner, coauthor of *Joy in the Journey*

"Alec Hill has been on the hero's journey into the valley that no one wants to visit but no one can avoid. This book reflects his vast gifts: an exceedingly learned and literate mind, a tenaciously thoughtful faith, and a rigorous commitment to honesty. It also contains gifts of the spirit: humility, gratitude, wonder, and acceptance. Reading it will bring healing to many, and wisdom to even more."

John Ortberg, senior pastor of Menlo Church, author of *Eternity Is Now in Session*

"Why should you read a book about cancer? Because four out of ten of us will get cancer in our lifetimes, and all of us will likely walk with a loved one fighting cancer. But you should read Alec Hill's new book for a different reason—because it is really about the precious gift of life. *Living in Bonus Time* will help you celebrate the life you've been given and maybe even reignite your sense of wonder and gratitude in the presence of the God who gives all of us life."

Richard Stearns, president emeritus of World Vision US,
author of *The Hole in Our Gospel* and *Unfinished*

"Rarely do you get the opportunity to witness someone walking through what would later become the contents of a book. I, along with others, have had the unique privilege of serving with Alec Hill prior to his diagnosis, of being arrested by the announcement of his diagnosis, of praying fervently during the time of his treatment, and of rejoicing in his recovery. As one whose younger brother and dear mentor were called by the Lord to himself through cancer, I celebrate Alec's 'living in bonus time' and the lessons that have come from it. Whether you are a cancer patient, cancer survivor, or caregiving friend or family of someone with cancer, this book's honesty, humor, and hope will bless you."

Claude Alexander, senior pastor of the Park Church, Charlotte, North Carolina, and past president of the Hampton University Ministers Conference

"Cancer lurks and devours lives every day. The diagnosis, treatment, and even post-treatment survival of cancer can be as life altering as the disease itself. Alec Hill knows this journey from the inside out. His candor, humility, faith, and love allow us all to peek in on this excruciating, mysterious, and all-too-common road. Whether cancer is our story or a loved one's, we are reminded again and again of the unexpected possibilities and realities of God's presence and grace, even on the cancer road."

Mark Labberton, president of Fuller Theological Seminary, author of *The Dangerous Act of Loving Your Neighbor*

"*Living in Bonus Time* is a candid and inspiring firsthand account of the life-changing impact of cancer. Alec Hill offers a comprehensive overview of his journey from diagnosis to remission, incorporating wisdom from the stories of others and prompting guided reflection. Whether you have been personally touched by the disease, are supporting a loved one, or are simply seeking a deepened perspective on life, this book will provide what you seek and more."

Santa J. Ono, president of the University of British Columbia

"With raw emotion and vulnerability, rich wisdom, and biblical truth, Alec Hill confronts some of the biggest challenges of our day—suffering, fear, and control. Through his own cancer story and the stories of others, he inspires us toward growth, even in the most difficult seasons of life. This book will minister to your heart!"

Tom Lin, president and CEO of InterVarsity Christian Fellowship/USA

"Cancer silences, frightens, and overwhelms. What Alec Hill does is give voice, courage, and strength to those in the midst of suffering and those who are caring for them. With the transparency and honesty of one who has been down in the pit, Alec's friendship and leadership in this space through *Living in Bonus Time* will strengthen many."

Sharon Cohn Wu, senior vice president at International Justice Mission

"Having survived the death of my twin sister after a fourteen-year journey with cancer, there are only two books I regularly recommend on cancer and grief and life. Now there are three. Alec Hill packs *Living in Bonus Time* full of not only his poignant personal story but also wisdom worth pondering, research worth knowing, quotes worth remembering, and stories of others that enlighten my own."

Anne Grizzle, family therapist and coauthor of *Treasures in Ashes: Twin Discoveries from a Cancer Journey*

"Alec Hill's engrossing story reminds me of how the Psalms include songs both of trial and tribulation, of victory and release. The Psalms were personal ('The Lord is my shepherd') and communal ('He heals all our diseases'). So Alec's story portrays both lament and recovery from disease as well as the terrible in-between times. It describes not just one person's courage but also how much we need each other, the power of community, when we go through life's dark passages."

Leighton Ford, president of Leighton Ford Ministries and author of *A Life of Listening*

"More than one in three people will get a cancer diagnosis at some point in their lives. Alec Hill is one of those people. His clear-eyed chronicle of this journey—from the anxiety and fear at diagnosis, to the pain and isolation of treatment, and ultimately the guilt and joy of recovery—is infused with his experience of God's presence throughout. Alec opens his life to us with honesty and integrity, wrestling with and trusting in a God who rarely provides neat answers. His story provides wisdom for anyone who has experienced suffering or questioned God's plan."

Denise Daniels, coauthor of *Working in the Presence of God* and professor at Seattle Pacific University

"Heart-stoppingly honest and beautiful at the same time! Alec Hill shares his journey with cancer and provides a thoughtful, deeply insightful engagement with the universal questions: Why me? Is God good? Who am I? Alec, informed by a life seasoned with habits of faithfulness, navigates the abyss with honesty. A helpful resource for anyone trying to respond to unexpected interruptions in life."

Nikki Toyama-Szeto, executive director of Evangelicals for Social Action at the Sider Center

"As I reflect on the cancer death of my best friend—as well as my own near-death experience—this book takes me on a journey of hope in the midst of profound loss, joy mingled with pain, and faith emerging from despair. *Living in Bonus Time* challenges us with unfiltered honesty to be more compassionate, kind, and resilient in the midst of suffering. Alec proves to be a faithful mentor as he draws from his own story."

Shaila Visser, global senior vice president, Alpha International and national director, Alpha Canada

LIVING IN

Surviving Cancer, Finding New Purpose

BONUS TIME

Alec Hill

An imprint of InterVarsity Press
Downers Grove, Illinois

InterVarsity Press
P.O. Box 1400, Downers Grove, IL 60515-1426
ivpress.com
email@ivpress.com

InterVarsity Press® is the book-publishing division of InterVarsity Christian Fellowship/USA®, a
movement of students and faculty active on campus at hundreds of universities, colleges, and schools
of nursing in the United States of America, and a member movement of the International Fellowship
of Evangelical Students. For information about local and regional activities, visit intervarsity.org.

All Scripture quotations, unless otherwise indicated, are taken from The Holy Bible, New International
Version®, NIV®. Copyright © 1973, 1978, 1984, 2011 by Biblica, Inc.™ Used by permission of Zondervan.
All rights reserved worldwide. www.zondervan.com. The "NIV" and "New International Version"
are trademarks registered in the United States Patent and Trademark Office by Biblica, Inc.™

While any stories in this book are true, some names and identifying information may have been
changed to protect the privacy of individuals.

Cover design and image composite: Cindy Kiple
Interior design: Jeanna Wiggins
Images: hourglass: © urfinguss / iStock / Getty Images Plus
        man silhouette against star background: © Mohaimen Wareth / EyeEm / Getty Images

ISBN 978-0-8308-4594-1 (print)
ISBN 978-0-8308-3500-3 (digital)

Printed in the United States of America ♾

InterVarsity Press is committed to ecological stewardship and to the conservation of natural resources in
all our operations. This book was printed using sustainably sourced paper.

Library of Congress Cataloging-in-Publication Data

Names: Hill, Alexander (Alexander D.), author.
Title: Living in bonus time : surviving cancer, finding new purpose / by Alec Hill.
Description: Downers Grove, Illinois : IVP, an imprint of InterVarsity
  Press, 2020. | Includes bibliographical references and index.
Identifiers: LCCN 2019041669 (print) | LCCN 2019041670 (ebook) | ISBN
  9780830845941 (paperback) | ISBN 9780830835003 (ebook)
Subjects: LCSH: Cancer—Patients—Religious life. | Hill, Alexander
  (Alexander D.) | Death—Religious aspects—Christianity.
Classification: LCC BV4910.33 .H54 2020 (print) | LCC BV4910.33 (ebook) |
  DDC 248.8/6196994—dc23
LC record available at https://lccn.loc.gov/2019041669
LC ebook record available at https://lccn.loc.gov/2019041670

P 25 24 23 22 21 20 19 18 17 16 15 14 13 12 11 10 9 8 7 6 5 4 3 2 1

Y   37   36   35   34   33   32   31   30   29   28   27   26   25   24   23   22   21   20

~ DEDICATED TO ~

Mary, my lifelong love,
incredible caregiver, and gifted editor.

———

Grant, my brother and donor, with whom I now share
not only faith but DNA.

———

Laura and Carolyn, beloved daughters who
jump into dark valleys with me.

———

Dr. Bart Scott, the oncologist who saved my life.
And to Drs. Nike Mourikes, Walter Longo, and Randall Roenigk,
who played key roles in my healing.

———

The infusion nurses, aides, and staff on the fifth floor of
the Seattle Cancer Care Alliance who sustained
(and loved) me for eighty-seven days.

———

The one hundred patients in the first bone marrow transplant trial
forty years ago, of whom only twelve lived a single year.

———

Chris Dolson, my pastor and dear friend.

———

Leighton Ford, my wise mentor.

———

Barry Crane, the friend who encouraged me to write this book.

———

Heidi Potter, Marilyn Rydberg, Jon Ball, Sharol Hayner, and Ken Elzinga—
loving caregivers whose spouses died far too young.

CONTENTS

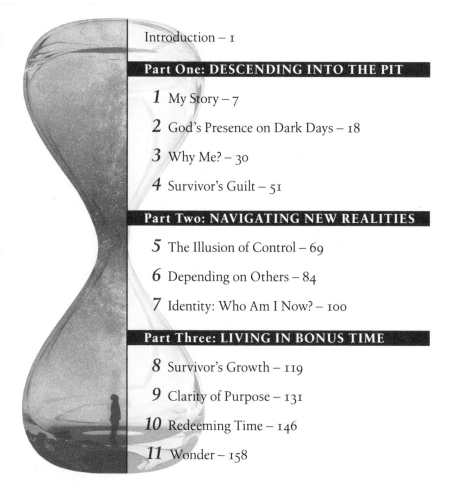

INTRODUCTION

F OUR OUT OF TEN OF US will be diagnosed with cancer during our lifetimes. This vile disease—with its incredibly diverse portfolio of manifestations—touches virtually every family.[1]

Today, there are more than five times the number of cancer survivors than just a half-century ago.[2] None of us asked to join this club, but we are grateful to still be alive. Although each of our stories is different, we share common fears and hopes. Profound questions arise: Why am I still here? Where is God in all this? Can anything good come out of my suffering? How should I live differently now?

Cancer changes us. Beyond the alterations to our bodies, we have the opportunity to learn profound spiritual lessons. Facing mortality, our assumptions, priorities, and behaviors are all open to change.

Bonus time is a metaphor borrowed from the sport of soccer. During ninety minutes of regulation time, the clock is not stopped for injuries, fouls, or substitutions (as in basketball). Instead, a designated referee mysteriously tallies all the breaks and then adds extra time. Players don't know whether the game will last another two or twenty minutes.

Cancer survivors live in metaphorical bonus time. We can point to a doctor's estimate of when our lives might have ended but did not (our regulation time). The additional months, years, or even decades we receive is not borrowed time—that implies something negotiated or loaned. Rather we live in bonus time, a season of grace.

How we live in bonus time matters. As survivors, we are stewards of a great trust. Not everyone gets the opportunity that we have—to have our souls reordered, to encounter God's presence in unique ways, and to serve others with remarkable motivation.

For the most part, the Lord has felt incredibly close through my various treatments. But, to be honest, there have also been stretches of deep confusion, incredible frustration, and intense sadness.

My hope in writing this book is to help you—my fellow pilgrims and your families—walk a perilous (and sometimes wondrous) journey. As a follower of Jesus, my reflections revolve around Scripture. In addition, while the narrative is rooted in my experience, profiles of others have been added to broaden the conversation. These are real people, many of whom I have known personally. Reflection questions at the end of each chapter encourage you to apply lessons learned to your own life.

A word to caregivers: you are my heroes. Thank you for the sacrifices you make. I hope this book honors the critical role you play. Far too often your needs are ignored as focus is placed on patients like me.

~ ~ ~

A brief note about myself. I was reared in Seattle by an amazing single mom and under the wings of two older brothers. In high school, I came to faith and attended (on scholarship) a remarkable private school that included the two future Microsoft founders. While in college, I volunteered for three years with Young Life at an urban high school. After law school, my regional World Relief team resettled one thousand refugees a year.

In my early thirties I became a professor and later a dean. My wife, Mary, and I reared two wonderful daughters. As a family, we enjoyed camping, reading, and the chronically bad Seattle Mariners baseball team. Unexpectedly, I was selected to lead InterVarsity Christian Fellowship/USA, a campus ministry based in Madison, Wisconsin. For fourteen frenetic years, I was part of an incredible missional community. We now reside back in the Seattle area.

~ ~ ~

The book is divided into three sections that mirror the emotional stages of most cancer survivors—downward, leveling out, and finally upward. First, in chapters one through four, we descend into the abyss. This includes being shocked by our diagnoses, walking with God through dark days, struggling with the theological problem of suffering, and facing survivor's guilt.

Second, in chapters five through seven, we adjust to our "new normal." Life stabilizes, but we are not quite the same people we once were. Forced to navigate new realities of control, dependence, and identity, we recalibrate expectations and relational dynamics.

Finally, in chapters eight through eleven we ascend into bonus time. As we get our sea legs back—moving from disequilibrium to balance—we are given the opportunity to experience survivor's growth, pursue deeper purpose, savor moments, and live with a greater sense of wonder. As counterintuitive as it may seem, cancer can transform us into better people.

PART ONE

DESCENDING INTO THE PIT

1

MY STORY

Chemotherapy is brutal. The goal is pretty much to kill everything in your body without killing you.

RASHIDA JONES

An individual doesn't get cancer. A family does.

TERRY TEMPEST WILLIAMS

Cancer is a wake-up call to remind us how high the cosmic stakes really are . . . and how short, brief, and frail life really is.

JONI EARECKSON TADA

Cancer is a disease of the genome. Mistakes in a cell somewhere in your body cause it to start to grow when it should've stopped.

FRANCIS COLLINS

E IGHT YEARS AGO, my doctor prescribed a variety of creams to reduce what appeared to be a common fungus familiar to most men—jock itch. Each product seemed to work for a while, but the rash continued to slowly spread. This went on for nearly a year. Finally, as my wife, Mary, and I prepared for a long trip, I asked to see a specialist.

Imagine my surprise when the dermatologist wanted to take a biopsy. "Down there?" I naively asked. After the procedure was conducted, I limped home.

A week later, while on a work-related trip, I listened to a message on my phone. "Mr. Hill," the dermatologist said in a flat voice: "You have an extremely rare type of glandular cancer. We haven't seen a case of Male Extramammary Paget's Disease (MEPD) in more than a decade." As I literally fell to the pavement, I recall him saying something about "removal."

Was this really happening? Sitting on the ground, I googled MEPD and read a scientific paper about the horrors experienced by men in Africa. Another article stated that my cancer was extremely rare with only five hundred cases reported worldwide annually. My reaction? Fear. Didn't glandular imply that the cancer would travel on my body's interstate highway? Might I lose a testicle . . . or worse? Could it spread to my brain? Might I die?

A few days later, I found myself as the primary subject of the "grand rounds" of the University of Wisconsin dermatology department. I understood this to mean that thirty doctors would examine me, trying to diagnose my rash and provide advice regarding next steps. Since a second opinion was needed, I reasoned, why not a whole team?

Who would have guessed that nearly half the observers would be female interns about my daughters' ages? As their little flashlights illuminated my private parts, any sense of modesty dissolved. I now better understand something of the indignity that women must feel during pelvic exams.

Not one of the specialists guessed my ailment. How could they? None had ever seen MEPD before. A tear glided down my cheek when I heard the consensus that I would not lose any body parts. I quietly thanked the Lord and held Mary's hand. What an incredible relief. But bladder, rectal, and colon cancer were still very much in play.

Through a providential connection at the Mayo Clinic in Minnesota, an appointment was made with a leading dermatological surgeon. There remained a very real risk that the cancer had spread to other parts of my body. For about a week, I struggled with the possibility of dying. Having only briefly brushed up against mortality in the past, I was totally unprepared for the emotions that poured out. It felt overwhelming.

After a scan showed no signs of the cancer spreading, I nearly jumped up and hugged the doctor. Even better, no radiation or chemo would be required. Still, the surgery lasted seven hours and required more than fifty stitches. That night I awoke in a hotel room, feeling something hot on my leg. The next day, the doctor seriously mulled the possibility of resewing the wound. I was horrified by the prospect. Thankfully, after hosting a lengthy consultation with a colleague (and waiting for the bleeding to stop), he decided it was unnecessary.

Three weeks in bed at home followed. At first, standing up and walking were difficult. I hurt. In particular, going to the bathroom was challenging. Eventually, I went back to the office, thankful that my altered private parts were not visible to the outside world. Within two months, strength returned and I was able to resume my precancer life. Little did I realize that this was but a prelude to the main event.

FAINTING SPELL?

Diagnosis. Fast-forward four years. As I bent down to grab yogurt out of the refrigerator, I blacked out and fell to the floor. Never having fainted before, I chalked it up to exhaustion after an eight-day trip on which I gave six talks in three cities.

Minimizing the incident, I made a conscious decision not to tell Mary. Why worry her? Of course, masked in this language of "marital care" was my fear of being grounded. My upcoming schedule, I rationalized, was simply too packed with important stuff to be interrupted.

A few days later, I shared what happened with my pastor and added that I had inexplicably lost seven pounds over the past few months. Looking at me with incredulity, Chris gave two pieces of advice I'll never forget: "First, always tell your spouse. And, second, never self-diagnose." He also let me know that if I didn't tell Mary, he would.

After appropriate groveling, I confessed to Mary. My penance was to see my general practitioner ASAP. He was unavailable, so an on-call physician examined me. Reviewing results from my blood test, she concluded, "You need to see an oncologist now." When she learned that there would be a seven-week delay in my appointment, she bypassed normal procedures and called the specialist's office herself to insist that I be prioritized. In doing so, this substitute doctor—whom I only met once—probably saved my life.

While describing my symptoms to the oncologist at the University of Wisconsin, I witnessed his mind clicking—weight loss, anemia, lightheadedness, decreasing energy, flu-like signs but no temperature. It was late Friday afternoon. Normally, he would have scheduled a bone marrow biopsy the next week with a nurse who specialized in the procedure. But, because he wanted the lab results immediately, he decided not to wait. Apologizing in advance for his heavy hands, he inserted a long needle into my hip, broke off a small piece of bone, and extracted it. Needless to say, it was a long ten minutes. His nurse held me down while I writhed in pain.

As we prepared to leave the office, the nurse gave me clear instructions to go to the hospital if I got sick over the weekend. When asked if her concern was related to possible infection from the procedure, she said no. She was worried about a compromised immune system.

The follow-up appointment was a shocker. The oncologist stated, "Mr. Hill, I have bad news. You have a cancer known as Myelodysplasia Syndrome (MDS). Your bone marrow is producing mutant white cells. If untreated, your immune system will fail, and you will die of a common cold within eighteen months. Its symptoms are similar to AIDS."

Swallowing hard, I asked, "Is it as bad as leukemia?" His response jolted me: "It's worse. There's only one possible cure—a bone marrow transplant. Of ten MDS patients, five will survive (defined as living two years, not exactly reassuring). Of those who live, three will have serious physical limitations. Only two will resume relatively normal lives." I later learned that notable MDS patients include TV anchor Robin Roberts (a survivor), astronomer Carl Sagan, and author Susan Sontag.

I imagined Mary living as a widow. I cringed at the prospect of informing our daughters, Laura and Carolyn, of yet another cancer. Death felt very close.

Second opinion. The next week Mary and I flew to Seattle for a second opinion. Half a century ago, bone-marrow transplants were pioneered at the Fred Hutchinson Research Center, so we knew we were in good hands.

Flying west, I journaled: "I've lived an incredible life. I wouldn't trade it for anyone else's. So, if the ride ends in the next eighteen months, I take great solace. I've loved deeply and been deeply loved." Despite the grim circumstances, I richly felt God's presence.

Entering the Seattle Cancer Care Alliance (SCCA) for the first time, my body involuntarily constricted at the smell of strange chemicals. David Scadden, professor of medicine at Harvard, aptly labels this foreign environment *Cancerland*. Questions popped into my mind: *Why are so many patients sitting alone? Will I become ashen like them? Why is it so quiet?* Scadden observes:

> A cancer diagnosis sends you into an alternative reality, Cancerland, where the usual things in life recede and it's easy to be overwhelmed by your condition, your treatment, and your prognosis. In Cancerland, you learn a whole new language . . . and you scan the horizon for signs of hope or danger.[1]

Following a round of lab work, my new oncologist placed me in a high-risk category. Of the ten thousand people who contract MDS annually, only five hundred have damaged third chromosomes. Extremely rare, *chrom-3* is regarded as chemo-resistant—horrible news since chemotherapy is central to the treatment.

My mind raced. Only five hundred people in the world? Can this really be happening again? Can lightning strike twice in the same place? Why me?

Since my cancer was so rare, SCCA doctors—despite being over-booked—opened a slot for me. Chrom-3 was both my curse and my ticket. Within three weeks, I resigned my position with Inter-Varsity, Mary prepped and sold our Madison condo, and we moved to Seattle. Every day, we were acutely aware of the monster lurking around the corner.

Transplant. The first order of business was to test my two brothers, Cy and Grant, to see if either was a bone-marrow donor match. The odds of a sibling match were 25 percent. If that failed, my oncologist would move to Plan B—the international donor pool. But the wait could take several months. Our daughters were by default only 50 percent matches.

Imagine our joy when Grant was identified as a perfect match. This also meant that my treatment would be expedited. Unlike MDS patients who rely on the international pool, I only had to endure a single month of pre-chemo shots to my stomach. When the nurse entered fully masked and gloved, I grasped the high tox-icity of the chemicals being injected. Over the next few days a burning red circle of inflammation tormented my flesh.

Mary and I moved into an SCCA apartment, our home for four months. It was an odd environment where seventy transplant pa-tients and their caregivers were told not to interact with each other. To prevent germs from spreading, there was no air-conditioning system. Though midsummer, we were instructed not to open our windows—it was critical to keep urban contaminants such as dust and mold out of the building. Sanitizer dispensers were hung on every floor.

For five days—after having a chest catheter surgically implanted—I received massive doses of chemo to kill all my white cells. On the day of full body radiation, with gallows humor, I chuckled when the radiologist said that I wouldn't be having any more children. At my age and stage, this comment was rather comical. But it also struck me that for women and men of child-bearing age, such news would be incredibly tragic. Blocking the estrogen that feeds their cancers or reducing the sperm count obstructs their ability to conceive children.

Grant's timeline and mine were handled independently but needed to merge on "day zero." As my blood counts plunged, he was being prepped by a separate medical team—a safeguard to avoid risking his health for my benefit. His goal was to produce five million stem cells. After receiving several shots, less than one million were harvested. The process was repeated a second day with the same results, providing only a total 1.7 million (37 percent of what was needed). Grant's platelet level dropped so low (from 195 to 40) that he needed a transfusion and could not give additional stem cells for several days. At age sixty-four, too much may have been asked of his body. Bone-marrow donors are typically young adults.

Thankfully, Grant's team had an ace up its sleeve—a $16,000 megashot. Feeling his body rumble, he didn't sleep much. The next day, he produced 2.2 million more units, bringing the total to four million. While less than optimal, my doctor said that it would have to suffice. The only other option was to shut down the transplant process and seek another donor from the international list. The risk of my decline in the ensuing months was simply too great to delay. Due to my treatments, I now had no functioning immune system.

Grant is a physical marvel—six feet four inches tall, 175 pounds. Prior to my transplant, he had biked across Iowa. But the procedure really beat him up, leaving him exhausted. Afterwards, his team counseled him to avoid any activity that might cause internal bleeding. His blood lacked the ability to coagulate properly. For the next six months, his white cell counts remained abnormally low.

The transplant itself was rather anticlimactic—more like a transfusion really. For four hours, Grant's stem cells dripped into my chest catheter. Fully conscious, I mostly read magazines.

For the next twenty-three days, while waiting for the transplant to graft, my white cell count was zero. Taking fifty pills a day, I became very ill. Scabs peeled off my radiation-fried body. Twenty pounds lost. Blood transfusions. Yellowish translucent skin. Incessant diarrhea. Insomnia due to steroids. It was truly a Job-like experience.

To minimize the risk of infection, Mary constantly sanitized every square inch of our apartment. Everything—bedding, towels, and clothes—had to be washed three times a day. She bathed me, changed the dressing on my chest catheter, monitored my medications, and cooked special meals. She was a saint. In virtual lockdown, we saw neither family nor friends.

As many cancer patients know, one of the side effects of receiving massive doses of poison is *chemo brain*. I couldn't read or complete sentences. All I could do was sit in a recliner, work on simple crossword puzzles, and watch TV.

For eighty-seven consecutive days, I was hooked up to receive infusions for up to four hours. While not painful, it was very awkward to use the bathroom. Tethered to a pole, I walked the clunky apparatus down hallways, always being careful not to tangle wires and tubes (one of which was screwed into my catheter). I wondered, *Is this hell?*

REFLECTION QUESTIONS

1. Describe a situation when you—or someone you love—was given horrific news. What phases did you go through emotionally? What questions did you ask God?

2. Reflect on Psalm 88. What does it say to you?

> LORD, you are the God who saves me;
>> day and night I cry out to you.
>
> May my prayer come before you;
>> turn your ear to my cry.
>
> I am overwhelmed with troubles
>> and my life draws near to death.
>
> I am counted among those who go down to the pit;
>> I am like one without strength.
>
> I am set apart with the dead,
>> like the slain who lie in the grave,
>
> whom you remember no more,
>> who are cut off from your care.
>
> You have put me in the lowest pit,
>> in the darkest depths.
>
> Your wrath lies heavily on me;
>> you have overwhelmed me with all your waves.
>
> You have taken from me my closest friends
>> and have made me repulsive to them.

I am confined and cannot escape;
 my eyes are dim with grief.
I call to you, Lord, every day;
 I spread out my hands to you.
Do you show your wonders to the dead?
 Do their spirits rise up and praise you?
Is your love declared in the grave,
 your faithfulness in Destruction?
Are your wonders known in the place of darkness,
 or your righteous deeds in the land of oblivion?
But I cry to you for help, Lord;
 in the morning my prayer comes before you.
Why, Lord, do you reject me
 and hide your face from me?
From my youth I have suffered and been close to
  death;
 I have borne your terrors and am in despair.
Your wrath has swept over me;
 your terrors have destroyed me.
All day long they surround me like a flood;
 they have completely engulfed me.
You have taken from me friend and neighbor—
 darkness is my closest friend.

2

GOD'S PRESENCE ON DARK DAYS

Nobody knows the trouble I've seen.

Nobody knows but Jesus.

NEGRO SPIRITUAL

Practice the Presence of God.

Above all, remember Him when you are in peril.

BROTHER LAWRENCE

Faith is the bird that feels the light and sings when the dawn is still dark.

RABINDRANATH TAGORE

Jesus' presence illuminates all darkness, enters through all locks,

and grants in the midst of prison the most pleasant freedom.

CATHARINA VON GREIFFENBERG

A S I ENTERED THE CANCER TUNNEL, many fears assailed me. These included worries about pain, possible physical limitations, and even death itself. But my greatest concern was something else: might the growing medical storm overwhelm my sense of God's presence? Might I be thrust into a "dark night of the soul"?

The phrase "dark night of the soul" was coined by John of the Cross, a sixteenth-century Spanish mystic. Mother Teresa described it as a "terrible sense of loss . . . this untold darkness, this loneliness, this continual longing for God."[1] Reformed scholar R. C. Sproul depicted it as "no ordinary fit of depression, but a crisis of faith that comes when one feels abandoned by him."[2]

I experienced the dark night once in my life. Following a broken romance while in college, a profound spiritual isolation and depression set in for more than a year. As I look back, the crisis was not so much about the failed relationship as about the cracking of my worldview. As a new believer I thought that I would be immune from pain if I obeyed God.

Consequently, when agony flooded my soul, I nearly lost my faith. For the only time in my life, I had suicidal thoughts. Like Jonah in the Old Testament, I ran from God, pleading aloud while hitchhiking on an isolated Wyoming road, "Where are you? Why have you left me so alone?" In the Psalms, David made a similar entreaty,

> How long, LORD? Will you forget me forever?
>> How long will you hide your face from me?
>> Do not turn a deaf ear to me.
> For if you remain silent,
>> I will be like those who go down to the pit.[3]

The dark night is a particularly ominous specter for cancer patients. Walking into the hellhole of chemotherapy, radiation, and surgery, we crave light, not darkness. We covet hope, not despair. The last thing we need is to sense God's absence. Having cancer is bad enough; feeling spiritually abandoned would only multiply our suffering.

ASSURANCE

Conscious of these anxieties, I asked the Lord for assurance of his presence. The first came as Mary and I flew to Seattle for a second opinion on my MDS cancer. During a stopover, I noted an email from an InterVarsity leader I was mentoring. Since only a handful of people knew of my diagnosis—and she was *not* one of them—I was stunned to read: "Alec—Greetings. I don't know all you are facing but this morning I was praying at 9:20 and felt the Lord say to remind you, 'Fear not, I am with you.' So, be encouraged that the Lord is with you!"

Standing in Terminal D of the Minneapolis-Saint Paul airport, I wept. What made her message even more astonishing was the fact that I had just selected Isaiah 43 as my sustaining Scripture. The parallels between her message and this passage are striking:

> Do not fear. . . .
> When you pass through the waters,
>   I will be with you;
> and when you pass through the rivers,
>   they will not sweep over you.
> When you walk through the fire,
>   you will not be burned. . . .
> For I am the LORD your God.[4]

Another assurance awaited in Seattle. While being prepped for my second bone-marrow biopsy, I reflected on how badly the first one had gone in Wisconsin. Entering the surgical room, I was sweating and my body was stiff as a board. But things took a surprising turn when a nurse named Grace introduced herself. I almost laughed aloud—her name symbolizes so much to me. As we talked, her faith became evident. She introduced her assistant, Dennis, who turned out to be a lay pastor (an amazing "coincidence" in secular Seattle). Under her gentle touch, my body relaxed, and I experienced a surprisingly low level of discomfort. An expert in pain management, she talked me off an emotional cliff.

Confirmation of God's presence also came through unexpected inner peace. During the forty-day post-transplant period—when I didn't know whether I would live or die—I journaled, "With Mary running errands, I could easily feel alone. But, instead, I'm feeling the thickness of your presence. You are here. If I were to die tomorrow, this is what I would enter into. And this is but a down payment. I love you so much, Father."

It later dawned on me that forty is a well-used number in Scripture, often depicting trials and uncertainty. Noah waited forty days before the floodwaters abated. Moses led the people of Israel for forty years in the wilderness. And Jesus was subjected to forty days of temptation in a dry place.[5]

Paradoxically, my forty days of uncertainty constituted one of the richest spiritual times of my life. Rereading the stories of Noah, Moses, and Jesus, I now realize that this was true for them as well. Photos show just how zombie-like I appeared—gaunt, jaundiced, and wasted. Yet somehow the Lord embraced me in an extraordinary way. While my exterior self was a mess (a fragile "jar of clay" as the apostle Paul puts it),[6] my interior self was quickened. In another journal entry, I reflected:

> Father, why am I so calm? So at peace? It's really rather remarkable and is clearly an act of your grace. To live is Christ and to die is gain. While I would rather live, I'm also excited about being with you soon. My mantra from the beginning has been "I trust you." It's surprising just how much I do.

I sincerely believed that I was being prepared for death—as if God were building a bridge to heaven. His presence became the common denominator between this life and the next. In the odd context of bodily torment, I experienced what ancient rabbis described as *Shekinah*—a physical place where God makes himself personally known. Our cancer apartment became a holy dwelling where the Lord met me. I experienced a surprising space of warmth, love, and wholeness. My fear of death abated as his presence calmed me and provided a deep peace. I was ready to go.

It is important for me to acknowledge that not every cancer patient has an experience like mine. Each journey is different. Some linger deeper (and longer) in the darkness of fear and isolation. But God sees us wherever we are and connects with us in unique ways.

PROFILE: STEVE HAYNER

For three decades Steve was my friend—as pastor, university colleague, and InterVarsity predecessor. A few years older, he was always a step ahead. When I needed counsel, Steve provided nonjudgmental wisdom. His kindness, brilliance, and joyful laugh were legendary to all who knew him.

While serving as president at a seminary near Atlanta, he was diagnosed with pancreatic cancer. The five-year survival rate of this horrible disease is 7 percent. Those who loved him feared the worst.

Over the course of the following year, Steve and his wife, Sharol, opened their lives via a blog. Posthumously, these reflections were compiled into a book, *Joy in the Journey: Finding Abundance in the Shadow of Death*. As his cancer spread, they did not sugarcoat his profound physical suffering. But they also wrote of God's closeness:

- "We are definitely in the fiery furnace from Daniel 3 but we are not alone. God's presence is very evident."

- "The Spirit of God is very present. This is a sacred journey where the distance between heaven and earth shrinks. . . . A place of shalom. I am so thankful."

- "God is the one secure place for my hope because it's not dependent on changing circumstances. How very freeing."[a]

Though Steve's earthly story ended quite differently than mine, we shared a common assurance of the Lord's presence in dark times and a deep confidence in eternity. Steve's courage and constancy in the face of death continue to impact my life.

[a]Steve Hayner and Sharol Hayner, *Joy in the Journey: Finding Abundance in the Shadow of Death* (Downers Grove, IL: InterVarsity Press, 2015), 27, 80-81, 103, 124.

GOD'S PRESENCE DURING CRISES

Why do many of us sense the Lord's presence most vividly during traumatic events? While counterintuitive, it is frequently in moments of great pain that fellowship with God is most intimate. Maybe it is because we are more attentive. Or perhaps when we have exhausted all human remedies, we turn to him in utter dependence. Jesus invites, "Come to me, all you who are weary and burdened, and I will give you rest."[7]

Before my cancers, I couldn't comprehend how persecuted believers maintain their faith in abominable situations. Now I understand that utter need elicits utter faith.[8] Life in the abyss motivates us to reach to heaven. There is nowhere else to turn. As Peter asked Jesus after many disciples deserted him, "To whom shall we go? You have the words of eternal life."[9]

While in prison, the apostle Paul was able to separate his *interior self* from his *exterior condition*. Reflecting on physical pain and isolation, he recognized that strength emanating from his spiritual core was not contingent on external circumstances: "Though outwardly we are wasting away, yet inwardly we are being renewed day by day."[10]

This is exactly what we are encouraged to do as cancer patients. Though suffering bodily, we are to seek God's strength in our interior selves. Church father Tertullian echoed Paul's words: "The body is shut in, but all is open to the spirit . . . it may roam abroad on the way to God. The leg does not feel the chain if the mind is in heaven!"[11]

GOD'S PRESENCE IN NORMAL TIMES

Troublingly, there is a tendency to relax spiritually when we are physically whole. We draw near to the Lord in a time of calamity but then slip back to a lukewarm status quo. Postcancer, when we are out of immediate danger, it is far too easy to lose a sense of urgency. We must heed Moses' warning as the people of Israel entered the promised land: "when you eat and are satisfied, when you . . . settle down, and when . . . all you have is multiplied, then your heart will become proud and you will forget the LORD your God."[12]

24

While the Lord remains constant and trustworthy, our tendency is to drift. C. S. Lewis compares our spiritual disposition to a tilted field on which balls continuously roll downhill, away from God.[13] A well-known hymn says it all: "Prone to wander, Lord I feel it. Prone to leave the God I love."[14]

Some believe that Shekinah experiences like my forty days are but a temporary grace given to those near death. I completely disagree. Once we've encountered his glory at a deeper level (even while in pain), we aspire for more. I treasure the rich spiritual moments I experienced during my slow-motion brush with death. Despite the wretched condition of my body, God's glory was life-giving, even oddly joyful. That time has become the benchmark of my spiritual life. Augustine aptly labeled it "the sweetness."[15]

Again, I recognize that each cancer journey is unique. Whatever your particular circumstances, I pray that the Lord's presence will give you light in a dark season.

SPIRITUAL DISCIPLINES

Followers of Jesus are encouraged to construct spiritual houses on rock so that when the rains come, the streams rise, and the winds blow and beat against us, we will not fall.[16] Cancer is like a Category 5 hurricane. Its powerful winds and driving rains batter us. We desperately need solid ground beneath our feet lest we tumble into total disequilibrium.

In other words, it is important—starting with small steps—to daily build our lives on the solid foundation of the Lord's presence. For those already in the pit of medical treatment, these may be very short steps indeed. As radioactive blue dye slowly dripped into my arm prior to a PET (positron emission tomography) scan for my first cancer, I lay alone in a dimly lit room. Rather than slipping into despair—imagining the worst-case scenario of cancer moving to my brain—I recited and meditated on Psalm 23 for an entire hour.

Memorizing the passage paid rich dividends that day. As I centered on the good Shepherd's nurture and provision, images of calm waters and cool pastures replaced the cold steel and plastic panels that surrounded me. My fears were hedged by the presence of an attentive Father. This led to an unexpected sense of calm, even peace. When my body entered the scanner, I was in a much better place emotionally.

Practicing spiritual disciplines is like digging a well. When crises hit, we are able to draw water for our soul's care. Healthy habits such as praying, meditating on Scripture, observing the sabbath, journaling, going on long walks, being part of a small group, taking retreats, singing spiritual songs, attending worship services, and being under pastoral care are all helpful practices.

To learn more about pursuing spiritual formation with greater intentionality, I recommend the writings of James Bryan Smith, Richard Foster, Ruth Haley Barton, and Dallas Willard.[17]

NOT FORMULAIC

There remains something marvelously mysterious about the Lord's presence. No five-step formula allows us to dictate the Spirit's movement. Having said that, Scripture describes a pathway forward. As we walk with humility and gratitude, we are to have "confidence to enter the Most Holy Place . . . [to] draw near to God with . . . full assurance."[18] Though we traverse through the valley of death—perhaps even dark nights of the soul—we are not alone. He does not abandon us.

For cancer pilgrims, this is good news on dark days.

PROFILE: BROTHER LAWRENCE—A MODEL FOR LIVING IN GOD'S PRESENCE

Poverty forced Nicholas Herman to join the French army. In 1636, his leg was seriously injured during a battle and he was discharged. Over the next few years, he sought God and was spiritually transformed.

Joining a Parisian monastery as a lay minister, he was given a new name: Brother Lawrence. For six decades, he humbly served his fellow priests by performing low-order tasks such as cooking, cleaning, and repairing sandals. But his acute sense of God's presence touched all who knew him.

Due to his piety, wisdom, and joyfulness, he became a highly influential spiritual leader in the community. After he died—and against his wishes—his teachings were published in a book titled *The Practice of the Presence of God*.

Four centuries later, his name produces nearly 700,000 hits on Google.[a] Why are so many fascinated by this obscure and disabled French monk? Why is his counsel still sought today?

Perhaps it's because we yearn to understand how he cultivated such a rich life with the Lord. Pain didn't deter him. Nor did his lameness. Even mundane work didn't interrupt his sense of being close to God:

I turn my little omelet in the pan for the love of God. . . . The time of business does not differ from the time of prayer. In the noise and clutter of my kitchen . . . I possess God in as great tranquility as if I were on my knees at communion.[b]

[a]Carmen Acevedo Butcher, "The Limping, Unceasingly Praying Brother Lawrence: How a 17th-century Cook and Sandal Maker Still Helps Us Practice the Presence of God," *Christianity Today*, September 2009, www.christianitytoday.com/history/2009/september/limping-unceasingly-praying-brother-lawrence.html.
[b]Brother Lawrence with Harold Myra, *The Practice of the Presence of God* (Grand Rapids: Discovery House, 2017), 1, 135.

REFLECTION QUESTIONS

1. Have you ever felt a keen sense of the Lord's presence during a crisis? If so, describe.

2. Have you ever experienced a dark night of the soul? If so, unpack your feelings. What are its lingering effects, both positive and negative?

3. Do you regularly sense the Lord's presence during "normal times"? If so, what spiritual disciplines move you in his direction? If not, what disciplines might help?

4. In Psalm 31, how does David seek God's presence from a dark place? What lessons can we learn from him?

> Be merciful to me, Lord, for I am in distress;
>   my eyes grow weak with sorrow,
>   my soul and body with grief.
> My life is consumed by anguish
>   and my years by groaning;
> my strength fails because of my affliction,
>   and my bones grow weak. . . .
> But I trust in you, Lord;
>   I say, "You are my God."
> My times are in your hands;
>   deliver me from the hands of my enemies,
>   from those who pursue me.
> Let your face shine on your servant;
>   save me in your unfailing love.
> Let me not be put to shame, Lord,
>   for I have cried out to you. . . .

How abundant are the good things
    that you have stored up for those who fear you,
that you bestow in the sight of all,
    on those who take refuge in you. . . .
Praise be to the LORD,
    for he showed me the wonders of his love
    when I was in a city under siege.
In my alarm I said,
    "I am cut off from your sight!"
Yet you heard my cry for mercy
    when I called to you for help.

3

WHY ME?

My God, my God, why have you forsaken me?

JESUS

Things fall apart. The center cannot hold.
Mere anarchy is loosed upon the world.

WILLIAM BUTLER YEATS

Lightning makes no sound until it strikes.

MARTIN LUTHER KING JR.

Within one year, my son was diagnosed with cancer,
my mother had five life-threatening hospitalizations,
my husband's dental office burned to the ground.

ANNE GRAHAM LOTZ

M Y ODDS OF CONTRACTING TWO UNRELATED CANCERS, each with only 500 cases reported globally per year, was 0.000000000000005 percent. This raises the simple question: *Why me?*

Most cancer patients have a bundle of similar queries. Is everything random? Why did we draw the short straw? Where is God in all this? Were we selected for some type of Job-like test?

For Mary and me, these questions became even more agonizing during the interval between my two cancers. Why was our youngest daughter shot in the head during a botched mugging?[1] The bullet came perilously close to entering Carolyn's brain, leaving a permanent three-inch ridge on the back of her skull. Losing 20 percent of her blood, she nearly bled to death. Seventeen metal staples were required to close the wound. The call from San Francisco General Hospital's emergency room was *the* most horrific moment of our lives. While she survived and subsequently recovered, answers are hard to find. *Why her?*

THEODICY

Human pain raises the age-old problem of *theodicy*: why does an all-powerful and good God allow suffering? Is it possible to hold to a belief in an intimate and almighty Father without accusing him of authoring evil?[2]

The word *theodicy* was famously coined by German philosopher Gottfried Leibniz in the eighteenth century. Claiming that we live in the "best of all possible worlds," he argued that a certain level of pain is necessary to balance the moral universe.[3] However, when a massive earthquake struck Lisbon on All Saints Day 1755, killing up to fifty thousand people—including thousands attending

Sunday mass—many asked how God could allow so much suffering to occur. In the face of such agony, Leibniz's highly cerebral (and exceedingly optimistic) theodicy floundered. Voltaire had a field day mocking him in the satire *Candide*.[4]

Countless subsequent attempts have been made to create tidy theodicies. Several of them will be explored in this chapter. But all fall short. Human suffering remains, in part, a mystery. We continue to ask: Why do babies die at birth? Why do innocents perish in war? Why do we contract cancer?

Scripture is not naive about suffering. Commencing in Genesis, it presents a complex tension of three parallel truths: (1) bad human choices, (2) chaos unleashed by these choices, and (3) God's sovereignty. While each concept is intrinsically complicated in its own right, the real difficulty comes when we attempt to harmonize them. Philosophers call this an *antinomy*—when apparently irreconcilable truths exist side by side.

A heads-up: in both substance and tone, this chapter is just plain difficult. Please stay with me. I promise less messy (and more hopeful) chapters ahead. But first, we must take a deep dive into the abyss.

BAD CHOICES

In the creation narrative, God made everything good.[5] Not only were human beings whole but nature flourished as well. No theodicy existed because everything was in harmony (*shalom* in Hebrew). Cause and effect worked simply. There was no cancer or death.

In granting free will, God gave humans the ability to choose good or evil. As rational agents, our first ancestors regrettably opted for the latter. Theologians refer to this as *the fall*. Martin Luther described resultant human nature as *curvatus in se*, curved in on itself—warped, self-deluded, and self-centered.[6]

Though distorted, our free wills remain operative today. If our decisions are good, we benefit physically and emotionally. But the opposite is also true. When we are gluttonous, we add weight. When we don't control anger or anxiety, our blood pressure rises. When we are intimate with multiple partners, we contract sexually transmitted diseases.

The cause-and-effect explanation of suffering is most clearly stated in early parts of the Old Testament. Those who obey the Lord will be fertile, prosperous, safe, and respected. On the other hand, those who don't obey will be poor, sick, unsafe, lonely, and oppressed. The New Testament echoes this teaching: "What is sown today will be reaped tomorrow."[7]

For cancer patients, however, this approach rings incomplete. Though the rationale that "bad choices cause suffering" explains some pain, it simply cannot explain all. For example, while it may connect the dots for 85 percent of lung cancer patients who smoke, what about the 15 percent who have never lit up?[8]

After my diagnoses, I worried whether any of my bad decisions had caused my cancers. For example, had swimming twenty times in a clogged and murky Russian pool somehow affected my cells? Before jumping in, I remember asking myself, *Is this safe?* Might I have absorbed some weird cancer-producing chemicals that bit me two decades later?

The simple reality is that the vast majority of our cancers can't be tied via a straight line to a particular bad choice. When asked whether my Russian escapade might have triggered either cancer, both of my oncologists categorically denied any causal connection. In other words, I didn't "merit" cancer because of a stupid decision.

In isolation, the cold logic of cause and effect leads to a horrific conclusion: we are to blame for our cancers. We must have done something to deserve them. This dodgy—and far too simple—karma-like approach is perilous on many levels.

In his Pulitzer Prize-winning novel *The Bridge of San Luis Rey*, Thornton Wilder illustrates the danger of utilizing cause and effect as a sole rule of thumb. After a Catholic priest witnesses five Peruvians plunge to their death when a footbridge collapses, he investigates their lives. Convinced that they must have been very bad people to merit such a cruel fate, he assigns one to ten points to each in categories of character, piety, utility, and age. However, as Wilder describes each of the victims, we see the utter futility of the priest's airtight theodicy. Morally, the dead are no better or worse than their surviving peers.[9]

While bad choices certainly contribute to suffering, they do not explain the totality of human pain. This is particularly true of most cancers. Clearly, a second (and supplementary) explanation is needed.

PROFILE: JERRY SITTSER

Professor Jerry Sittser led an idyllic life—a loving and creative wife, four vibrant children, and a wonderful job. After a lovely afternoon in Idaho, the family was driving home to Spokane on an isolated road at twilight when a drunk driver struck their van. In an instant, three generations of women—his mom, wife, and four-year-old daughter—perished. The driver's wife died as well.

In his book *A Grace Disguised*, Sittser reflects:

I remember the realization sweeping over me that I would soon plunge into a darkness from which I might never again emerge as a sane, moral, believing man. . . . All I wanted was to be dead. Only the sense of responsibility for my three surviving children and the habit of living kept me alive. . . . I was tortured by the question of where God was that night. Would I ever be able to trust him again?

As Sittser began to rebuild his life, he experienced deep joy in his surviving children. But even then, the nightmare didn't end. Unable to prove whether the drunk driver or his wife was at the wheel at the time of the crash, the culprit was acquitted in a jury trial.[a]

[a]Jerry L. Sittser, *A Grace Disguised* (Grand Rapids: Zondervan, 1995), 126.

CHAOS

The fall unleashed a second stream of suffering. While I confess to not understanding exactly how it works, it is impersonal, universal, and random. Unconnected to cause and effect, it wreaks havoc. Family members die in auto accidents, mutant cells rebel inside our bodies, and children are haphazardly shot. The perfect, peaceable, and orderly world of Eden is long gone. The apostle Paul writes that creation itself "groans" under its crushing weight.[10]

Tragically, no one is exempt. Distributed in a nonlinear and unpredictable way, bad things happen to villains and innocents alike.[11] Jesus taught that rain falls on the just and unjust, just as weeds grow side by side with wheat.[12] That the good can and do die young is exemplified by the death of my six-year-old cousin after he was sucked out his family's van by a tornado. This unimaginable event occurred two decades ago and the family has never fully recovered.[13]

Such randomness is deeply disturbing. Sociologist Émile Durkheim labels this sensation *anomie*, a French word meaning disorderliness.[14] When life doesn't work as we perceive it should, we experience frightening disequilibrium. It pierces our false sense of confidence that we control more than we actually do.

When diagnosed, I complained to God. Why were seemingly "bad" people able to glide through life untouched while I got repeatedly smacked? Sure, I'm far from perfect, but am I worse than they are? This is a profoundly unsettling mystery. Psalm 73 echoes my sentiments:

> I saw the prosperity of the wicked.
> They have no struggles;
>   their bodies are healthy and strong.
> They are free from common human burdens;
>   they are not plagued by human ills. . . .
> They clothe themselves with violence. . . .
> [A]lways free of care, they go on amassing wealth.
> Surely in vain I have kept my heart pure
>   and have washed my hands in innocence.
> All day long I have been afflicted,
>   and every morning brings new punishments.[15]

Something sinister grabbed my body and twice submerged it. The primary image of this awful randomness in the Old Testament is the ocean's turmoil.[16] It is as if a massive and irresistible wave dragged me down and nearly killed me. Simone Weil, a French mystic, observes, "Affliction is anonymous. . . . It is the coldness of this indifference—a metallic coldness—that freezes all those it touches right to the depths of their souls."[17] The fallen world is an unkind place.

When Cambridge professor Norman Anderson was asked how he could retain faith even though his wife was suffering from dementia and all three of his children had predeceased him, he responded: "I don't ask 'why me?' No. But I do ask the question, 'why not me?' People of faith are not immune to this world's ills. Like all fallen creatures, we die in airplane crashes, suffer cancer, and lose children."[18]

From the third chapter of Genesis onward, Scripture portrays human suffering as normative—not only for bad guys but for saints like Joseph, Job, Jeremiah, and James.[19] In particular, the books of Job, Psalms, and Ecclesiastes teach that some suffering is disconnected from specific moral failings. The psalmist repeatedly rues the fact that the blameless suffer, and God rebukes Job's acquaintances for their facile karma-like conclusion that his agony is merited.[20] Likewise, Ecclesiastes laments the fact that cause and effect are not always in sync and that the innocent experience randomness:

> The race is not to the swift
>> or the battle to the strong,
> nor does food come to the wise
>> or wealth to the brilliant
>> or favor to the learned;
> but time and chance happen to them all.

Moreover, no one knows when their hour will come:

> As fish are caught in a cruel net,
>> or birds are taken in a snare,

so people are trapped by evil times
   that fall unexpectedly upon them.[21]

In the New Testament, Jesus taps directly into this flow of thought. When asked by his disciples why a man was born blind (implying fault for a bad choice), Jesus replied: "Neither this man nor his parents sinned."[22] In other words, it was completely wrong-headed to draw a causal link between the blind man's genetic disorder and any moral misconduct by family members.[23]

And when a tower randomly crushed eighteen people, Jesus asked rhetorically, "Do you think they were more guilty than all the others living in Jerusalem? I tell you, no!"[24] In other words, direct cause (sin) and effect (pain) played no role in their deaths. Rather, as part of a broken world, chaotic things can happen to anyone at any time. In these passages, Jesus refutes the tidy theodicy expressed by Thornton Wilder's fictitious priest.

Over the years, I've observed that my African friends have less difficulty accepting suffering as normative than I do. Taking randomness as a given, they worry less about the *why* and focus more on helping others. But as an American boomer, I've imbibed a Disneyesque worldview—there will always be a happy ending. Of course, this is a myth. Recently, I was surprised to learn that Walt Disney never allowed the word *death* to be used in his presence, fervently avoiding funerals (including his brother's). Attempting to shut out the world's chaos, he created parallel universes.[25] In doing so, he rejected Augustine's wisdom that "mortal life is harsh."[26]

Lament. As cancer patients living in a fallen world, we sometimes simply need to release the sheer awfulness of it all. Being targeted by an indiscriminate malady is horrible. When fear gripped me, I wept, complained, and even screamed. I recall going into our basement and putting a pillow over my mouth to mute my cries of agony.

Lament is the brackish water—neither salt nor fresh—where our polarities meet: doubt versus faith, anger versus submission, withdrawal versus pleading. It's the place where we shriek against chaos and the pain it inflicts. When truly bad things happen, we need space to let out our unfiltered emotions. It is a place without easy answers, rational explanations, or quick fixes—an odd combination of grief, rage, confusion, and a desire to be rescued.[27] Daniel Simundson, an Old Testament scholar, observes, "Lament allows us . . . the freedom to admit even bad theology and hostile thoughts."[28]

In my carefully written video to InterVarsity staff announcing my bone-marrow cancer and resignation, I departed from the script at one point to spontaneously add, "It's okay to say that this sucks. It really sucks." This became the most remembered line of my eight-minute talk. Why? Because it resonated with everyone's sense of lament. Raw, honest, and unbridled, it expressed a shared sense of confusion, sorrow, and frustration. It gave everyone permission to emote honestly—not to hide behind a mask of false stoicism.[29]

Ecclesiastes reminds us that there is "a time to weep . . . a time to mourn."[30] Jesus' cry from the cross—"My God, why have you forsaken me"—is the ultimate lament. If the Son of God could be so candid—and not sin—so may we.[31]

Many cultures—such as Korean, Kenyan, and Cambodian—audibly lament together in times of great pain. Likewise the African American church. But, I must confess, I've observed much less of this in the white church, where congregational lament seems to be a largely forgotten spiritual practice. With a book titled "Lamentations" and up to 40 percent of the psalms fitting into this genre, it is hard to grasp how this practice has been so neglected.[32] Nancy Duff, a Princeton Seminary professor, reflects:

> Lament allows us to speak from the darkest regions of the heart, where our despair threatens to overwhelm us. In so speaking, we do not exhibit a lack of faith, but stand in a biblical tradition that recognizes that no part of life, including the most hideous and painful parts, is to be withheld from God.[33]

PROFILE: JONI EARECKSON TADA

At age seventeen, Joni dove into Chesapeake Bay. Misjudging the depth of the water, she hit bottom far too quickly. Her backbone splintered, and she became a quadriplegic, paralyzed from the shoulders down. During lengthy physical therapy, she grew suicidal.

Learning to paint with a brush in her teeth was a first step back from the abyss. As voice recognition software became available, she started to write books, record albums, host a radio program, and even appear in a movie about her life. A ministry to the disabled, Joni and Friends, slowly evolved. Over the past four decades, she has impacted millions globally. An early advocate of the Americans with Disabilities Act, she has also influenced public policy.

In her forty-eighth book, *The Healing Place: Wrestling with the Mysteries of Suffering, Pain and God's Sovereignty*, Joni reflected on the problem of theodicy. Experiencing horrific back pain, she lamented:

> Why has God allowed this? I'm almost sixty years old! Why such agony and distraction at this point in my journey, after all these years

of enduring, preserving, and seeking to serve him? Even though multitudes of devoted, good-hearted Christians pray in great faith, many eyes will stay blind. Many babies will die at birth. Many cancers will not be eradicated.[a]

At age sixty-one, Joni was diagnosed with stage 3 breast cancer and underwent a mastectomy. She continues both to question God and to follow him. She admits that it is often an uneasy journey.

[a] Joni Eareckson Tada, *A Place of Healing: Wrestling with the Mysteries of Suffering, Pain, and God's Sovereignty* (Colorado Springs: Cook, 2010), 26.

GOD'S SOVEREIGNTY

Thankfully, the biblical narrative doesn't end in despair. Our bad choices and the resultant chaos are not the end of the story. Rather, immediately after the fall, God introduced a redemptive pathway for us through a promised Messiah. Isaiah prophesied that this redeemer—though a "man of suffering"—would bring healing and hope to the world. He would "take up our pain" and "bear our suffering." David predicted that he would be forsaken by God, mocked, and tortured.[34]

The biblical concept of incarnation—that Jesus came from heaven to earth to suffer with and for us—is unique among world religions. Tim Keller tells of an Australian Muslim who reacted adversely: "'How preposterous that the creator of the universe should be subjected to the forces of his creation—that he would eat, sleep, and go to the toilet—let alone die on a cross.' To which the Christian speaker responded: 'What the Muslim denounces as blasphemy, the Christian holds precious: God has wounds.'"[35]

Why did I—and countless others—incline toward God when I was in pain? Because through Jesus, he has suffered too. Can any of us claim pain approximating the brutal torture of a Roman crucifixion? Or the even more intense agony of separation between the Father and Son?

Years after the death of his family members, Jerry Sittser reflected:

> The God I know has experienced pain and therefore understands my pain. In Jesus, I have felt God's tears . . . and witnessed the redemptive power of his suffering. . . . He is not aloof but draws near to me when I suffer. He is vulnerable to pain . . . and acquainted with grief. God is a suffering sovereign who feels the sorrow of the world.[36]

When we hurt, God doesn't walk away. Rather, he stands in solidarity with us because he loves us. "Only a suffering God can help," observed Dietrich Bonhoeffer.[37] This was certainly my experience on deeply dark days. Though wildly disoriented, I leaned more heavily upon him. And he was there.

God's unknowable side. Unlike most religions, Christian Scripture reveals our heavenly Father in a highly personal manner. He loves, gets angry, and forgives. He is portrayed as a good shepherd, gracious spouse, and righteous judge.[38] Particularly in the coming of Jesus, we see the divine character on full display. The Messiah entered our world and became subject to its postfall chaos. Why? To redeem us. The gospel is called *good news* for a reason.

But another side of God's being is simply beyond us. We can't read his mind or plot his actions. To try to understand why he restores some to health and not others is to enter a great mystery. We simply don't know. Anyone who claims to fully comprehend God's thoughts on such matters is either self-deluded or a liar.

Why did Jesus tell Peter that he would die but his fellow apostle John would live: "If I want him to remain alive until I return, what is that to you?" Why did the apostle Paul's "thorn in the flesh" (a painful and recurring disability) persist? Why did Isaac and Jacob go blind? Why were John the Baptist and the apostle James executed? Why, according to the writer of Hebrews, were saints tortured, flogged, enchained, stoned, sawed in two, and decapitated?[39]

We simply don't know. Jeremiah compares God to a divine potter and humans to clay.[40] Contemplating this metaphor, Paul asks, "Who are you, a human being, to talk back to God? Shall what is formed say to the one who formed it, 'Why did you make me like this?'"[41] As cancer patients, we have to be careful not to overstep our bounds by insisting on full answers to our *why me* questions. Tim Keller reflects, "While God's ways are as opaque to us as a parent's are to an infant, still we trust that our heavenly Father is caring for us. . . . If God were small enough to be understood, he wouldn't be big enough to be worshipped."[42]

Living with this unknowable sense of God's ways pushes some people away. But others, like Jerry Sittser and Joni Eareckson Tada, have come to peace with it. As have I. Job persisted in not denouncing God despite immense misery and loss.[43]

How we respond to apparently random suffering like cancer marks a great dividing line. Some opt for faith. Others opt out— either losing their faith entirely or seeing God as heartless and mean-spirited (labeled "misotheism" by philosophers).[44] Why our good God heals some—like me—and not others is *the* unanswerable question. He alone is sovereign. Like you, I find this mystery to be both terribly frustrating and incredibly humbling.

Max Lucado tells an insightful story of famed botanist George Washington Carver. Born a slave, Carver was both deeply pious and incredibly inquisitive. In his journal he recorded the following prayer:

> "Oh, Mister Creator," I cried out, "why did you make this universe?"
>
> And the Creator answered, "You want to know too much for that little mind of yours. Ask me something more your size."
>
> So, I said, "Dear Mister Creator, tell me what man was made for."
>
> Again, He spoke to me and said, "Little man, you are still asking for more than you can handle. Cut down the extent of your request and improve the intent."
>
> Then I asked my last question. "Mister Creator, why did you make the peanut?"
>
> "That's better," the Lord said.
>
> And He gave me a handful of peanuts and went back with me to the laboratory, and together we got down to work.[45]

Rejecting the health-and-wealth gospel. Perhaps the most tantalizing aspect of our redemption is its "now, but not yet" nature. In the "now," we experience the Lord's forgiveness and rich presence. Some of us are even healed. For the most part, however, it is obvious that we are "not yet" living in complete *shalom* (wholeness and flourishing). Rather, we dwell in a chaotic place where cells mutate and tornadoes kill. Full restoration will come only after death.

This is where the so-called *health-and-wealth gospel* goes awry. A recent construct that has spread globally, it claims that the kingdom of God has fully arrived. Presented as a self-evident theodicy, it promises that if we live righteously, everything good in life will come our way—including robust health. This *realized eschatology* (emphasizing "now" and deleting "not yet") sees all of God's blessings as guaranteed to us right now, in this life.

Like karma, the health-and-wealth gospel promises immunity to suffering if we live uprightly. Cancers will not touch us. Bad bosses will not affect us. Abusive spouses will not harm us. God becomes our personal genie who resolves all our problems. But this theology totally disregards the stream of biblical teaching in Job, Psalms, and Ecclesiastes—and later affirmed by Jesus.

This sense of divine-human reciprocity—a contractual quid pro quo formula of my obedience in exchange for his protection and abundance—is a one-way ticket to confusion and heartbreak. As a college student, this false teaching led me into a very dark place, leaving me depressed and nearly causing me to lose my faith.

When calamity occurs, as it inevitably will, such erroneous ideas are incredibly dangerous. In the rich soil of perceived injustice—when we see entitlements unfilled—seeds of resentment easily bloom into bitterness toward God. I can't imagine entering the cancer tunnel holding such beliefs. It's a train wreck in the making.

Beware of false messengers. Six weeks before my transplant, so weakened by chemo that I was unable to stand, a well-meaning couple approached me at a reception. Declaring that it was God's will for me to forgo the transplant—doctors are unnecessary—they warned me not to be disobedient. Steeped in the health-and-wealth gospel, they admonished me to exercise greater faith. If I were to suffer or die, their theodicy would place the blame directly on me.

I became so angry that I almost lashed out but was too emotionally and physically fragile to do so. I just crumpled back into my chair as I watched them walk away. Like Job's counselors, they thought they knew the mind of God but were, in reality, false prophets.[46]

Joni Eareckson Tada tells a similarly horrific story of a stranger named David. Approaching her in a church parking lot, he confidently declared that it was God's will to heal her. After delivering a canned minisermon, he concluded: "Joni, you must have a lack of faith. I mean, look at you. You're still in your wheelchair!"[47]

At times, sufferers simply want quiet empathy, not armchair advice. In his poignant book *A View from a Hearse*, Joseph Bayly reflects on two men attending his wife's funeral.

> I was sitting, torn by grief. Someone came and talked to me of God's dealings, of why it happened. Of hope beyond the grave. He talked constantly, he said things I knew were true.
>
> I was unmoved except to wish he'd go away. He finally did.
>
> Another came and sat beside me. He didn't talk. He didn't ask leading questions. He just sat beside me for an hour or more, listened when I said something, answered briefly, prayed simply, left.
>
> I was moved. I was comforted. I hated to see him go.[48]

Full restoration awaits. In Scripture, the closing chapter of human history commences with the resurrection of Jesus. Celebrated at Easter, it is central to the Christian faith. Paul declares that we too will one day receive new bodies that are imperishable, glorious, and powerful.[49] Likewise, John foresees a time when God "will wipe every tear from their eyes. There will be no more death or mourning or crying or pain, for the old order of things has passed away."[50]

The good news is that our battered, broken, and aging bodies will one day be fully restored. As I look at my scars and feel my aches, I long for a new day of full agility and energy. No more cancer. No more arthritis. No more pain.

Joni Eareckson Tada also longs for that "not yet" day:

> I want to encourage us to look up from day-to-day battles to focus on that time of ultimate healing awaiting us. The times when every eye will be opened, the ears of all those who are deaf will be unstopped, the tongues of those who cannot speak will shout for joy, and the lame will leap like deer. Oh, what a glorious day that will be![51]

PROFILE: SANDY FORD

Leighton and Jeanie Ford were awed and perplexed by their eldest son. Sandy's burning intensity was off the charts; his devotion to God profound. As a highly competitive high school runner, he literally left everything on the track, once collapsing as he crossed the finished line.

At age twenty-one, Sandy experienced a forty-minute heart arrhythmia. Rushed to the hospital, electroshock stabilized him. After conducting a battery of tests—and evaluating his heart surgery from three years earlier—doctors concluded that another operation was necessary.

Leighton recalls, "I cried to the Lord out of the depths. . . . It just hurt all over." He asked God, "For what reason wouldn't you heal him? I know you can. If you won't heal my son, you must be something different from what I always imagined." Tragically, the doctors could not restart Sandy's heart postsurgery.[a]

Now in his eighties—nearly four decades after Sandy's death—Leighton writes, "There really is no fix for such grief, is there? No neat way to describe it or deal with it, simply because its edges are ragged."

He looks forward to seeing his son in heaven and realizes the mystery of retaining—even growing in—faith amid such circumstances: "My heart was broken. But my faith held, or rather it held me." Quoting the Irish poet John O'Donohue, he reflects: "Beauty is not all brightness. In the shadowlands of pain and despair, we find slow, dark beauty."[b]

[a]Leighton Ford, *Sandy: A Heart for God* (Downers Grove, IL: InterVarsity Press, 1985), 111-43.
[b]Leighton Ford, *A Life of Listening: Discerning God's Voice and Discovering Our Own* (Downers Grove, IL: InterVarsity Press, 2019).

Close to God even in pain. Karl Marx famously called religion the "opiate of the masses."[52] By promising better things to come, he claimed, people are numbed to their present pain. However, it is certainly arguable that his alternative—no hope beyond the grave—is far darker. Did Jerry Sittser, Joni Eareckson Tada, and Leighton Ford lessen the quality of their lives by exercising faith?

In truth, walking closely with God has given them hope instead of despair, meaning rather than nihilism. Three years after the accident, Jerry Sittser reflected, "The tragedy pushed me toward God, even when I did not want him. And in God, I found grace, even when I was not looking for it. . . . All I could do is let God love me in my misery."[53]

I confess to not fully understanding how the threefold antinomy of choice, chaos, and sovereignty intersects vis-à-vis human suffering. Harmonization of these truths often seems impossible. In many situations, *Why me?* remains a mystery and the problem of theodicy unresolved. Tim Keller wisely summarizes:

> There is no fully satisfying theodicy that completely shows why God is justified in allowing evil. Nevertheless, the Christian doctrine of the resurrection and . . . renewal . . . comes the closest to any real explanation we have. . . . Someone might say, "But that's only half an answer to the question." Yes, but it is the half we need.[54]

REFLECTION QUESTIONS

1. How has suffering affected your life?

2. Describe a time you lamented.

3. Have you been able to trust God through your suffering (or that of a loved one)? If so, explain.

4. In Psalm 13, how does David guide us to think about suffering?

> How long, LORD? Will you forget me forever?
>   How long will you hide your face from me?
> How long must I wrestle with my thoughts
>   and day after day have sorrow in my heart?
>   How long will my enemy triumph over me?
> Look on me and answer, LORD my God.
>   Give light to my eyes, or I will sleep in death,
>   and my enemy will say, "I have overcome him,"

and my foes will rejoice when I fall.
But I trust in your unfailing love;
 my heart rejoices in your salvation.
I will sing the Lord's praise,
 for he has been good to me.

4

SURVIVOR'S GUILT

The problem with surviving is that you end up with the ghosts
of everyone you've left behind riding on your shoulders.

PAOLO BACIGALUPI

My biggest challenge? Without a doubt,
survivor's guilt. I try to deal with it by helping others
as much as I can, but I want to do more.

GWEN, STAGE 4 COLON CANCER SURVIVOR

Guilt is to the spirit what pain is to the body.

EDGAR BEDNAR

Oh my friends, my friends, forgive me that I live and you are gone.
There's a grief that can't be spoken; there's a pain goes on and on.

MARIUS, "EMPTY CHAIRS AT EMPTY TABLES"
IN *LES MISÉRABLES*

O N THE TWENTY-FOURTH DAY after my bone-marrow transplant, my white-cell count reappeared for the first time, a sign that my brother's cells were starting to graft. Though only 30 (4,000-10,000 is normal), it was a welcome harbinger of things to come. The next day, it was 250. Then 360 and 440. I had the incredible sensation that new life was taking root in my body. Hundreds of Grant's cells were exponentially turning into thousands. Soon they would turn into millions and billions. I was slowly being resurrected.

On the fortieth day—after my third bone-marrow biopsy—my oncologist said, "Mr. Hill. I have good news. You have 100 percent of your brother's white cells and no traceable cancer cells. You now have a 90 percent chance of living." Mary and I held hands and rejoiced. Really? Out of the woods? Life ahead?

From that date forward, I challenged myself to regain strength by walking. Wearing latex gloves, I slowly climbed a flight of stairs in our cancer apartment building. It was difficult—and I paused often—but each subsequent day got a bit easier. In time I was able to climb all six floors. Fatigue was slowly transformed into renewed strength. Within two months, I was walking up hills. My stamina, appetite, and weight all gradually returned.

Eventually, daily infusions ceased. Appointments became less frequent. Finally, on the hundredth day post-transplant, we were cleared to go home. It was an amazing experience to sleep in our own beds again. For the next eight months I lived in quasi isolation (jokingly referred to as "house arrest"). No church. No restaurants. No animals. No live plants. No little kids. No hugs. Apart from Mary, human contact was restricted to outside and at arm's length.

Why so many precautions? My new immune system was immature—I lacked the internal resources to fight infection. Flu and colds were a real fear. More significantly, the transplant had wiped all my childhood immunization shots. It was a full two years—730 days—before I received my final live virus shot.

WHY ME? PART 2

About six months into my recovery, I was once again confronted with the question *why me?* But this time it had a different significance. Why was I going to live while many of my peers were either dead or dying? Sitting in an oncology waiting room, I recall grilling God about a patient with three young kids: "Why am I well and she is sick? I'm past my prime; she's in her twenties. I have adult children; hers are still dependent."

Circling back to the *why me* question caught me off-guard. I never expected it to reappear as a surprise bookend to my cancer experience. No one had warned me about this uninvited guest. Unwittingly, I had bumped into survivor's guilt.

At the very time that I should have been thrilled by my trajectory—after all, only one in five bone-marrow transplant survivors lives without serious health limitations—I fell into a mild depression. For three months, perplexing melancholy descended on me like a damp shroud. Lethargy and sadness characterized my moods. Not every day. Not every hour. But a certain heaviness of spirit was undeniable. I sought counseling. A fellow cancer survivor aptly describes this sensation: "I was born into an incredible family. I had access to the best care. I married the kindest man alive. But why am I not overjoyed? I feel guilty about feeling guilty. Where do I go from here?"[1]

UNPACKING SURVIVOR'S GUILT

The American Association of Cancer Research defines survivor's guilt as the living wondering why others with whom they shared a common traumatic experience have perished. Often, we blame ourselves simply for being alive: "Why am I still here instead of them?"[2]

The syndrome was first identified among Holocaust survivors.[3] *Sophie's Choice*, a film about a mother who outlives Auschwitz after her two children are swallowed up by Nazi evil, captures the horrific trauma. In recent decades, psychologists have expanded the definition to include soldiers who lose buddies in war and survivors of near-death situations. On the one-year anniversary of a mass shooting at a Florida high school, a nineteen-year-old suffering from survivor's guilt—her best friend had perished—took her own life.[4]

It is now recognized that nearly half of all cancer patients experience survivor's guilt.[5] My first cancer produced no such adverse feelings. After a clean bill of health following surgery at the Mayo Clinic, I quickly moved on with life. Three months later, I was healthy and rarely looked in the rearview mirror.

But my bone-marrow cancer was completely different. Why? Two factors came into play. First, I was housed with seventy other transplant recipients. This created an unspoken bond, a community of shared suffering. Though warned not to interact for fear of infection, we pulled for each other. When two apartment units unexpectedly were vacated, we knew this meant that patients had died. Without telling me, Mary regularly checked mailbox names. One afternoon, she observed a neighbor being wheeled out on a gurney by medics to the hospital where he soon died.

Our shared experiences produced a remarkable sense of tribe. Only those in the "club" knew what it was like to have spinal taps, radiation scabs, chemo sickness, and chest catheters. Notes a medical professional:

> Survivor's guilt makes little sense to someone who has not sat with fellow patients in the waiting room, compared diagnoses, and received encouragement. . . . But to a cancer survivor, it makes perfect sense. Patients gravitate toward one another. They may have the same type and stage of cancer and yet have very different outcomes. Because of that tight bond, they are more inclined to feel a sense of survivor's guilt.[6]

Second, the imminence of death—theirs and mine—was powerful and inescapable. Sick and failing people surrounded us daily in elevators, infusion bays, and blood-draw rooms. While it is now easy in retrospect to regard the cancer ward as a place of healing, at the time it often seemed like the exact opposite—a "voyage of the damned."[7] This shared suffering made it incredibly painful to lose "one of our own."

PROFILE: BILL AND JOAN

A month after Mary and I moved into cancer housing (room 203), Bill and Joan became our next-door neighbors (room 204). Since he and I shared the same cancer (MDS) and we were all Christians, the four of us connected rather quickly despite a shared need for isolation. A caring and fun person, Joan brought life to a sad place. For Halloween, she fetched decorations from home to embellish the lobby and championed a door-decorating contest. Drab portals became places of artistic creativity. Small stuff, but hope-building.

Bill's medical story differed markedly from mine in that it took nine months from diagnosis to transplant. Finding a suitable donor consumed valuable time. When a young European was finally identified, Bill's "blast count" (an increase in bad cancer cells) jumped into unsafe territory. Receiving monthly chemo shots to bring this count down, he was almost ready on several occasions.

So, to Bill and Joan's relief, his blast count finally stabilized and a transplant date was set. Tragically, a week before his procedure, he contracted a simple cold and was admitted to the hospital. With a severely compromised immune system weakened by months of chemo, the cold quickly developed into pneumonia. Unable to fend off the infection, he died two days later.

His death hit Mary and me hard. We deeply mourned Joan's loss. MDS patients have a 50 percent survival rate. Never have I experienced a statistic so personally. Room 203 lived. Room 204 died.

Meanwhile, I continued to sail through the process. The juxtaposition of these events—Bill's death and my good health—produced deeply conflicting emotions. On the one hand, I was thankful for the grace of God in my life for a miracle in slow motion. My strong cell counts, regained weight, reduced medications, physical stamina, and increased mental acuity were amazing.

On the other hand, Joan packed her belongings to go home and start a new life without her best friend of thirty-five years. Why was Bill gone and I still alive?

I now understand that survivor's guilt is normal. But at the time, its impact left me feeling isolated and unable to articulate what was going on inside. It was certainly a tangle of complex feelings.[8] A breast-cancer survivor recalls weeping over a badly cooked pan of eggs:

I'd had cancer for God's sakes, and I was crying over eggs? I was supposed to be a survivor. . . . We survivors are supposed to be happy and grateful, to embrace our second chance at life. . . . I felt worthless and guilty. How did I have the right to feel sadness? People died of cancer, and I didn't. . . . Survivor's guilt is real.[9]

POSTTRAUMATIC STRESS DISORDER

Our youngest daughter, Carolyn, underwent extensive posttraumatic stress disorder (PTSD) counseling the year after she was shot. As I described my symptoms to her, she encouraged me to get help. Psychologists now include survivor's guilt as a symptom of PTSD. Four indicators stand out.[10]

First, sufferers reexperience traumatic events via upsetting memories and feelings of distress. A slow release of hidden, dark memories occurs in the brain. This lapse of time is actually a grace from God. If we had to absorb all the pain at once, it would probably be overwhelming. So, our brains are wired to store bad memories until we can cope. As we heal, these recollections gradually filter into our consciousness. I must confess, however, that it was no fun reexperiencing traumatic events just as I was beginning to feel better. Tragically, many turn to alcohol or drugs to deaden the refreshed pain.

Second, negative feelings choke us like invasive weeds. As we turn inward and withdraw, our motivation to engage life diminishes and energy ebbs. We become numb and mired in sadness, guilt, and anxiety. Though my symptoms were less dramatic, the heaviness of my soul was certainly real. Sadly, others go much deeper into the pit. Jamie Hutchings, a childhood cancer survivor, writes, "By 15, it all came crashing down. I was depressed. By 17, I was suicidal. I felt guilty to be alive. I had watched some of my friends die from the same leukemia. If I turned on a movie where the child was dying, chances were high that they were dying of leukemia."[11]

Third, survivors may become edgy, irritable, and lose concentration. In Judith Guest's book (and Oscar-winning movie) *Ordinary People*, a family tries to cope with the loss of a teenage son in a sailing accident. The surviving younger brother, who was also on the boat, struggles with mood swings, insomnia, and anger. He fails at school, seeks counseling, and considers suicide. His mother (played by Mary Tyler Moore in the movie) appears to be strong—not pursuing outside help—and criticizes his "weakness." Only as the plot unfolds do we realize that the son's reactions are normal and her stoicism is not.[12]

Finally, survivors may try to avoid anything that might trigger memories of the trauma. This includes emotional withdrawal, evading conversations, and dodging specific places. But grief cannot be bypassed, hospital waiting rooms cannot be sidestepped, and loved ones cannot be excluded. Withdrawal leaves us alone at the exact time we need to be embraced. A spouse laments:

> My husband was diagnosed with Hodgkin's Lymphoma. Within two months, his best friend was also diagnosed. After going to each treatment side by side, his friend passed. . . . My husband has kept busy with lots of events, fundraisers, and the creation of a 501c3 organization, but hasn't taken time to accept the loss of his friend. He has shown signs of severe depression and was even admitted to a hospital.[13]

We heal most quickly when we acknowledge our grief. Simply punting our pain down the field is unhelpful. Jerry Sittser advises that the "quickest way to reach the light of day is not to run west, chasing after the setting sun, but to head east, plunging into the darkness until one comes to the sunrise."[14]

Having said that, there is no single timetable that works for all. Walking through past trauma is highly individualistic. Each of us is wired differently.[15] There is no shame in pursuing help when we feel something is wrong inside us. Looking back, I am a bit surprised by how proactive I was in asking for a professional counselor. It proved to be a significant step forward in addressing my confusion and pain. Simply being told I was not an outlier was a comfort.

CAREGIVER TRAUMA

Survivors aren't the only ones who experience trauma. For caregivers whose loved ones receive outpatient treatment—such as my first cancer—the emotional effects may be limited. But for those on the other end of the spectrum, duties assumed may be complex, burdensome, and long-term.

With my second cancer, Mary felt an intense fear that she might negligently cause my death by failing to kill every single germ. This sense of hypervigilance, which continued for two years, made it impossible for her to completely relax. Her quest to prevent infection became (using her words) "a compulsion." Likewise, she could not permit herself to get sick. Due to my lack of immunity, a simple sore throat would compel her to leave our residence.

Mary moved into self-preservation mode. Not able to focus on her own needs, she developed a sense of detachment. When friends asked how she was doing, her response was always the same: "Don't ask me how I feel. Ask what I'm doing." She now describes that time as "going clinical," putting her emotions on hold. "If anyone pricked my bubble, I feared that I would implode. My resolve, self-control, and strength might bleed out." Being a stoic helped her cope with a life-and-death situation. However, in the process, she gave up much of her personal identity and emotional balance.

As my healing progressed, Mary gradually evolved from being a *Caregiver* (capital C) to a *caregiver* (lowercase c) and then back to a *partner*. She began to rediscover a new sense of self. Stronger as a person (and in her faith), she is now finding new outlets for service and exploring a new chapter of life. I am eternally grateful for her sacrifice.

PROFILE: WAYNE AND HEIDI POTTER

I spotted Heidi's thick binder across the blood-draw waiting room. Recognizing it as the same notebook I had received fourteen months earlier, I surmised that she was a newbie. As our conversation commenced, her husband joined us. It turned out that Wayne, not she, was the patient.

The three of us hit it off immediately. I learned that his bone-marrow transplant was scheduled in a few weeks. A fifty-nine-year-old engineer, he had never been sick in his entire life. His oncologist was optimistic, giving him an 85 percent chance of recovery. Phone numbers were exchanged and a remarkable friendship ensued. Nearly daily, Wayne and I talked on the phone, texted, or emailed. Hope permeated each conversation.

Shortly after his transplant, however, the calls stopped. It was evident that something had gone horribly wrong. Concerned that I hadn't heard from him, I reached out to Heidi. She emailed that Wayne's skin was jaundiced and he was noticeably weakening. Mary and I prayed daily. Finally, after ten days of silence, Heidi called: "Wayne died a few hours ago. The transplant didn't kill him. Chemo toxicity did. It destroyed his liver."

> I fell to the floor and sobbed. Why Wayne? Why did the treatment meant to save his life kill him? Later, I learned that 2 percent of patients react as he did to poisonous drugs.[a]
>
> I recall numbly stumbling through Wayne's funeral. My head was in a fog. Hugging Heidi, I didn't know what to say. Why was I—older and with lesser odds—still alive and he was gone?

[a]M. O'Brien, "Mortality within 30 days of Chemotherapy: A Clinical Governance Benchmarking Issue for Oncology Patients," *British Journal of Cancer* 95, no. 12 (December 18, 2006): 1632-36.

SURVIVOR STEWARDSHIP

Is it possible to transform survivor's guilt into something constructive? Can feelings of remorse and sadness be redirected into acts of compassion? Is it possible for distress to serve as a motivator to do good for others? Can the loss of our friends—like Bill and Wayne—stir us?

Survivor's stewardship inspires us to care for those currently in pain. For me, this means reaching out to cancer patients, acting on their behalf as friend, servant, and advocate. Nearly every month, I converse with someone who is in the belly of the beast. The best way to manage survivor's guilt is to love others. As Jesus said, "to whom much has been given, much will be required." "Give, and it will be given to you."[16] By investing our lives in others, our pain is repurposed and our suffering redeemed.

Medical professionals stress the importance of redirecting our suffering for the benefit of others. Bradley Zebrack, a professor at the University of Michigan (and himself a Hodgkin's lymphoma survivor), labels it a "reframing of priorities": "In my interviews with patients, many say they feel guilty, but ultimately talk about a more positive—and potentially transformative—existential experience of determining what reasons they have to go on living. . . . They work in honor of others."[17]

Michael Levin survived lung and brain cancer as well as a heart attack. When his sister was diagnosed with cancer, he provided care until she died. Since then, he has served other patients through his local hospital: "You feel like you're making yourself worthy of the efforts that doctors, technologists, and nurses made on your behalf."[18]

Kindness can also be shown in the normal ebb and flow of life. Sandra Gahm, an ovarian cancer survivor, was waiting in an oncologist's office one day when she noticed a new patient. The woman was so nervous that she was unable to complete a simple medical questionnaire. When Sandra offered to play scribe, the woman was deeply appreciative.[19]

PROFILE: MARK CHARLES

As a seventeen-year-old, Mark drove his brother north from Navajo land to attend their grandparents' fiftieth anniversary in Denver. Near Santa Fe, Mark passed another car, hit a sign, and flipped.

His brother died instantly, and Mark suffered a serious head injury. His life was saved by off-duty medical professionals (a doctor, nurse, and emergency medical technician) who were driving south on the same road. Mark has no memory of the accident or the preceding hour.

Over the next four years, Mark disconnected emotionally. He never wept. Nothing unlocked his PTSD-protected brain. Not the first anniversary of the accident. Not visiting the site of the accident. Not going to the junk yard to see his wrecked car. Family and friends assured him that "it's not your fault." But, since it was a single-car accident, he thought, *Of course it was my fault.*

As a UCLA sophomore, he began to date a woman—the first person he had cared for since the accident. "The emotions freaked me out," he told me. "Guilt flooded in. I was convinced that God was going to kill me." The surge of pain became so overwhelming that he dropped out of school.

At a ministry retreat, a leader asked if anyone needed prayer for forgiveness. Realizing that he had never forgiven himself, Mark stood. Soon, he found himself prostrated on the floor: "It felt like a watermelon was being dragged out of my stomach, through my lungs and out my mouth. As I wept, I sensed Jesus holding me, emptying my guilt, pain, and shame. It was one of the most beautiful things I've ever experienced."

Twenty-five years later, Mark reflects, "I came to the point where I could live with myself again. The healing journey has taken years."[a] Today he advocates for Native American concerns in truth and reconciliation. His favorite Scripture is Isaiah 43.

[a]Phone interview with Mark Charles.

MOVING FORWARD

Survivor's guilt is real but need not be debilitating. Through counseling, journaling, and receiving care from others, our guilt can be transformed into a redeeming grace. Pain can be rechanneled to help others in need. Likewise, caregivers should not shrug off their own trauma but rather pursue outside expertise and community support.

Developing a sense of empathetic care for others is one of cancer's "gifts." I am clearly a better person for having known Bill and Wayne. The apostle Paul captures the concept well, encouraging us to steward hope and love (rather than guilt and sadness) to others:

"The God of all comfort, who comforts us in all our troubles, so that we can comfort those in any trouble with the comfort we ourselves receive from God. . . . If we are distressed, it is for your comfort. . . . Just as you share in our sufferings, so also you share in our comfort."[20]

RESOURCE: AMERICAN TRAUMA SOCIETY

If you are struggling with survivor's guilt or any form of PTSD, the American Trauma Society provides helpful resources, including support groups. These small groups are designed to ease feelings of stress, isolation, loneliness, and sadness. Each is facilitated by a trauma survivor and has access to a health professional. Most meet monthly.[21]

REFLECTION QUESTIONS

1. Have you ever experienced survivor's guilt? Or have you ever known someone who has? Discuss what it was like.

2. Describe a situation when your personal pain was converted into something positive. What process led to this repurposing? Did you feel that your suffering was redeemed (at least partially)? Explain.

3. Reflect on Isaiah 43:1-5, 7. In what ways does this passage apply to your life?

> Do not fear, for I have redeemed you;
> > I have summoned you by name; you are mine.
> When you pass through the waters,
> > I will be with you;

and when you pass through the rivers,
   they will not sweep over you.
When you walk through the fire,
   you will not be burned;
   the flames will not set you ablaze.
For I am the LORD your God,
   the Holy One of Israel, your Savior . . .
[Y]ou are precious and honored in my sight . . .
   I love you. . . .
Do not be afraid, for I am with you. . . .
[You are] called by my name,
   whom I created for my glory,
   whom I formed and made.

PART TWO

NAVIGATING
NEW
REALITIES

5

THE ILLUSION
OF CONTROL

Suffering shatters the illusion of self-mastery.

DAVID BROOKS

I can't always control my body the way I want to, and I can't control when I feel good or when I don't. I can control how clear my mind is. And I can control how willing I am to step up if somebody needs me.

MICHAEL J. FOX

Worrying does not empty tomorrow of its troubles:
it empties today of its strength.

CORRIE TEN BOOM

We can't control the current of events.
We can only float with them and steer.

OTTO VON BISMARCK

T HE PHRASE "ILLUSION OF CONTROL" was first used by psy-
chologist Ellen Langer to describe a form of self-delusion. It
occurs when we overestimate our ability to influence events.
Studies show that when people select their own lottery numbers,
they believe that they have a greater chance of winning than those
randomly selected by computer. Likewise, gamblers throw dice
harder when they want high numbers and softer for low numbers.[1]
My eldest daughter, Laura, believes that I can adversely impact the
fate of our favorite baseball team by prematurely claiming victory.

A comical example of illusory control involves traffic lights in
New York City. Installed in the 1970s, signs instructed pedestrians
to "push button and wait for walk signal." Fifteen years later, the
system was computerized and pushing a knob had no effect
whatsoever. However, the city neither replaced the mechanisms
nor informed the public. To this day, pedestrians continue to
push the buttons, presuming that they control the lights. Similarly,
in elevators installed after 1995, the "door close" feature works
only via a key.[2]

My illusion of control was shattered by cancer. A classic Type A
personality, I elbowed my way through life. And for the most part
it worked. Due to my proactivity, I enjoyed promotions and acco-
lades. But cancer wasn't something I could plan around. Or will
myself around. It was simply there—a formidable and nasty ad-
versary. Push the button as often as I might, the light was never
going to change. The elevator door was not going to close.

As I began to take stock of my puniness vis-à-vis cancer, I realized that much of my life had been built on a fiction. The chilling
reality was that I never had as much control as I presumed. I didn't
control being born an American white male boomer (four words

loaded with privilege). Neither did I control my brother Cy qualifying for a scholarship at an elite private high school. The fact that I followed as a legacy sibling allowed me to be classmates with an incredible group of young men.

The isolation of my post-transplant year afforded ample time to reassess this assumption. It was painful to realize that after asking *why me?* in terms of suffering, I had never asked it in terms of the benefits in my life. Rather than being humbly thankful, I proudly took credit for all *my* accomplishments. I adored the rewards of merit.

This false confidence created an inflated sense of control. In doing so, I unconsciously echoed the sentiments expressed in William Henley's famed poem "Invictus": "I am the master of my fate, I am the captain of my soul."[3] Though a Christian who should have known better, I took inordinate delight in my achievements and the recognition that followed.

But here's the harsh reality. I had no control over contracting cancer, finding a matching donor, or dictating how my body would react to copious quantities of poison. Henri Nouwen notes, "In the face of great pain or inescapable grief, we realize how little we control our lives, how feebly our protests change reality."[4]

I am now embarrassed by my lifelong habit of ascribing far more influence to myself over events than I actually possess. Rather than being captain of a large boat on a small lake, I am more akin to a man on a small raft in the Pacific Ocean. As such, I am a poster child for the *illusion of control*. Tim Keller captures how cancer opened my eyes:

> Suffering transforms our attitude towards ourselves. It
> humbles us and removes unrealistic self-regard and pride. It

shows us how fragile we are. . . . It does not so much make us helpless and out of control as it shows us we have always been vulnerable and dependent on God. Suffering merely helps us to wake up.[5]

PROFILE: STEVE JOBS

Steve Jobs created what biographer Walter Isaacson calls a *reality distortion field*. "Just as Star Trek aliens frame their own world through sheer mental force," Isaacson writes, "in Jobs' presence, reality was malleable." An Apple designer observed, "Steve was a force of nature with an indomitable will to bend any fact to fit the purpose at hand." Under his leadership, project teams produced an incredible flow of amazing breakthrough products.

Jobs believed that normal rules didn't apply to him. Rather, he viewed himself as a Nietzschean Übermensch, a superman able to control reality. If facts didn't suit him, he simply ignored them.

This grand sense of self caught up with him when, at the age of forty-eight, oncologists found a tumor on his pancreas. Dismissing their advice to pursue immediate surgery, he developed his own treatment plan that included visiting a psychic, trying alternative treatments found on the internet, and purging himself of "negative energy."

Isaacson says, "This was the dark side of his reality distortion field—his assumption that he could will things to be as he wanted." A member of Apple's board remembers "pleading with Steve every day" to have the surgery; "He had such a strong desire for the world to be a certain way that he willed it to be that way. . . . Sometimes it doesn't work. Reality is unforgiving."

Tragically, by pursuing his own course of treatment, Jobs wasted nine months before following his oncologists' counsel. But by then it was too late. Cancer had spread throughout his body. Likely, he would be alive today had he yielded control to his doctors earlier.[a]

[a]Walter Isaacson, *Steve Jobs* (New York: Simon & Schuster, 2001), 117-24.

CONTROL OVERREACH

The apostle James critiques those of us who try to control the uncontrollable:

> Now listen, you who say, "Today or tomorrow we will go to this or that city, spend a year there, carry on business and make money." Why, you do not even know what will happen tomorrow. What is your life? You are a mist that appears for a little while and then vanishes. Instead, you ought to say, "If it is the Lord's will, we will live and do this or that."[6]

Control overreach represents the height of human arrogance. Like Adam, Eve, and the builders of the Tower of Babel, we presumptuously overstep our bounds when we claim too much power. Before starting MDS treatment, I tried to overcontrol the situation by battering my medical team with one question after another even though there was only one treatment option. My excessiveness was abruptly squelched when a nurse named Jon slammed his fist on the table in frustration: "Damn it, Mr. Hill, are you going to trust us or not?"

Like Steve Jobs, I was looking for alternatives and trying to dictate the situation. Jon's reaction proved to be a turning point. From then on, rather than trying to tinker in the engine room as part of the crew, I accepted the fact that I was a passenger on the cancer boat.

A counterexample to my boorish conduct is provided by a former colleague of mine named Alex Anderson. Following the apostle James's advice, Alex prefaced his statements with a humble "if the Lord wills" multiple times a day. At the time, this felt like an annoying habit to me—akin to adding "uh" to each sentence. Now, however, I understand. Alex grasped the fact that he exercised only modest control over external circumstances and that he leaned into God's sovereign arms. Tragically, one evening while on a quiet walk, he suffered a heart attack and died in his late forties.

That many things lie beyond our control is evident merely by scanning the daily news—war, recessions, earthquakes, hurricanes, mudslides, fires, and floods. Consider the South Sudanese farmer who just a few years ago was celebrating the independence of a new nation. Today, he struggles in a Ugandan refugee camp. Or witness the plight of a Syrian public schoolteacher whose peaceful existence and fulfilling vocation was tragically ripped apart by a brutal civil war.

Less dramatically and closer to home, our cars malfunction, children misbehave, bosses get ornery, and jobs are discontinued. Trying to impose control over that which is uncontrollable is not only futile, it also creates stress and isolation.[7] Fifty million Americans experience panic attacks, phobias, or anxiety disorders each year. Stress-related illnesses cost $300 billion annually in doctor bills and lost productivity. Interestingly, on average, residents of other nations experience only one-fifth of our level of anxiety.[8]

The biblical Greek word for worry—*merimna*—connotes a divided mind. Max Lucado notes: "Worry takes a meat cleaver to our thoughts, energy, and focus."[9] A clinical therapist concurs: "Many people who enter my office with depression, anxiety, and stress-related issues have one thing in common: They spend a lot of time focusing on things they can't control. Rather than controlling their emotions, they're always trying to control the environment—and the people in it."[10]

Besides hurting ourselves, control overreach causes collateral damage. For example, those who express road rage over their inability to command traffic often lash out at others. Micromanaging bosses make life miserable for their staff. Overreaching parents harm the marriages of their adult children. Franklin Roosevelt's mom was so controlling that, when he first married, she bought side-by-side homes and knocked out a wall so she could enter at any time. Even after he became president, she threatened to cut him off from the family wealth if he displeased her in any way. Over time, her daughter-in-law Eleanor grew understandably resentful.[11]

CONTROL UNDERREACH

Recognizing the dangers of overcontrol, we must be careful not to swing too far in the other extreme. For cancer patients, undercontrol means becoming passive. Symptoms include failing to ask questions or pursuing a second opinion. Over time, feelings of powerlessness, depression, and even fatalism emerge.[12]

This equally unhealthy space—devoid of personal agency—is an easy place to drift when we are picked, poked, and prodded. Research indicates that dogs receiving ongoing electric shocks eventually learn helplessness: they lie down quietly and no longer respond to stimuli.[13] In our most depressed moments, we may be likewise tempted to acquiesce—losing confidence in our ability to change anything.[14]

As cancer survivors, we must be vigilant. Being inert (or detached) is not the solution and can be every bit as noxious as control overreach. While it may not be easy to cope with our altered bodies, physical limitations, and complex medicine regimes, it is important to diligently fight off despair. Lapsing emotionally, mentally, or spiritually is a dangerous path. Exits out of this trap include physical therapy and counseling.

A final word: being fully compliant with doctors' orders is quite different from exercising undercontrol. While it is always prudent to keep our eyes and ears open, at a certain point we must decide to trust the professionals who care for us.

APPROPRIATE CONTROL

Once our *illusion of control* bubble pops, we are free—perhaps for the first time in our lives—to assess our vulnerabilities with unclouded eyes. Careful not to swing wildly to passivity, we seek the healthy middle ground of *appropriate control.* In the Bible's very first chapter, God delegates dominion to us. While this authority has limits, we are charged as stewards to be proactive and creative.[15]

Four critical attitudes are essential for cancer survivors— *humility, trust, gratitude,* and *rest.* I confess to being better at describing them than living them out. Woven together, they produce balance and beauty.

Humility. Jesus blesses those who are "poor in spirit."[16] In meekness, we are encouraged to acknowledge that we are not little gods who control all that goes on around us. That results in narcissistic chaos. Rather, we are encouraged to concede that we are limited created beings who rely on—and take refuge in—an infinite and good God.

As people affected by cancer, we recognize that there are many factors that are simply beyond our control. Like the apostle James, we acknowledge our inability to foresee the future or to influence many aspects of our medical journeys.

PROFILE: MARTIN LUTHER KING JR.

When Dr. King was only twenty-six years old, he learned a life-changing lesson about humility and trust. After fellow clergy selected him to lead the Montgomery bus boycott and the effort began to succeed, he started to receive regular death threats. Late one night, while alone in his kitchen, a caller said he would bomb King's house and kill his family if he didn't leave the city within three days.

Dr. King's initial reaction was to try to control the situation: "I sat there and thought about a beautiful little daughter who had just been born. She was the darling of my life. . . . And I started thinking about a dedicated, devoted, and loyal wife who was in the next room asleep."

Next, exemplifying poverty of spirit, he humbly confessed his fears, "I bowed down over that cup of coffee. I prayed out loud that night, 'Lord, I'm weak now. I'm faltering. I'm losing my courage.'"

As he prayed aloud, his trust grew. He heard the Lord say: "Martin Luther, stand up for righteousness. Stand up for justice. Stand up for truth. And lo I will be with you, even until the end of the world. . . . I heard the voice of Jesus saying still to fight on."

That night transformed Dr. King's life. Assured that God would be his refuge, he went to bed peacefully. No longer worried about death, he rested not in his own control but in the sovereignty of God. Secular historians label this event "the kitchen prayer." While recognizing that a different man emerged that evening, they are unable to explain what happened in his soul.

People of faith understand that Dr. King encountered God in such an incredible way that he decided to trust no matter what came next. By relaxing his grip on control, he gained an inner confidence that the world could not comprehend. When his house was bombed three days later, a few of his angry parishioners threatened revenge. After calming them down, he sent them home.[a]

[a]David Garrow, *Bearing the Cross: Martin Luther King, Jr., and the Southern Christian Leadership Conference* (New York: Perennial, 1986), 57-60.

Trust. In the Sermon on the Mount, Jesus teaches extensively about the importance of trust and the danger of worry:

> Do not worry about your life. . . . Look at the birds of the air; they do not sow or reap or store away in barns, and yet your heavenly Father feeds them. Are you not much more valuable than they? Can any one of you by worrying add a single hour to your life? . . . Your heavenly Father knows that you need them. But seek first his kingdom and his righteousness. . . . Do not worry about tomorrow.[17]

While birds are active—they make nests and feed their young—they have no control over nasty storms and lurking predators. Yet Jesus says that God knows and provides. As cancer survivors, our posture is to be one of trust. We are not to stress today about what *might* happen to our bodies tomorrow. Why? Because the Lord is present. In his wisdom, Jesus knew what we need to hear. Providing comfort and hope, he assures us how precious we are to the heavenly Father.

In saying this, we do not close our eyes to the mystery of theodicy. Indeed, our suffering may very well continue. John Stott wisely counsels, "Jesus does not promise that believers are immune to all misfortune. Birds fall to the ground and get killed. His promise was not that they would not fall, but that this would not happen without God's knowledge."[18]

While I don't pretend to always understand the Lord's ways, I continue to trust him. Such faith isn't easy. But neither is it blind. Built step-by-step over years of walking with God, I've learned that he is indeed trustworthy. Two weeks after my MDS diagnosis—while still in a deep fog—I told the InterVarsity staff: "A lifetime of faith has taught me to expect to see his redemptive purposes in six, twelve, eighteen months. I firmly believe that he will somehow bring good out of this awful situation. He has done it so many times in my life."[19]

And, as my future hung in the balance during forty days of post-transplant limbo, I journaled: "Faith is patient, persistent, non-entitled, difficult, and rewarding. My mantra is I trust you. It's surprising just how much I do."

Gratitude. An emotional bull of a man, the apostle Paul struggled with control overreach most of his life. Competence and pride marked his early years. And yet, toward the end—suffering from ill health, rotting in jail, and being mostly abandoned—he moved to a remarkable place of contentment.

Despite appalling circumstances, Paul was grateful. One of his final letters, Philippians, contained not a single word of complaint.[20] Rather he wrote, "Rejoice in the Lord always. . . . [W]ith thanksgiving, present your requests to God. . . . I have learned to be content whatever the circumstances."[21] In this short epistle, he used the word *rejoice* six times, *joy* five times, and *thanks* thrice.

How was this possible? What was his secret to being joyful under such miserable circumstances? Rather than focusing on his horrific context, Paul concentrated on knowing Jesus and sharing the gospel. He was simply too thankful to be overwhelmed by demons or death.[22]

This is not to be confused with the power of positive thinking (yet another expression of overcontrol). "Though outwardly wasting away" and enduring "momentary troubles," Paul was grateful. He did "not lose heart" but was "renewed day by day" as he internalized an "eternal glory that far outweigh[ed]" his suffering.[23] As Max Lucado observes: "Thankfulness sucks the oxygen out of worry."[24]

Earlier, I introduced my friend Steve Hayner who died of pancreatic cancer. The title of his book, *Joy in the Journey: Finding Abundance in the Shadow of Death*, speaks volumes about his attitude during his final year of life. As it became apparent that his death was imminent, he reflected, "Every day, I ask myself how I should be using the gift of this day. . . . My call is to . . . be filled with hope, love, faith, and joy."[25]

Research indicates how critical gratitude is as a healing agent. David Desteno, a professor at Northeastern University, lists it as the first quality of emotionally healthy people. His studies demonstrate that an attitude of thankfulness changes us from the inside out, equipping us to make a positive difference even when facing adverse circumstances.[26]

I confess that gratitude doesn't always come easily for me. Having unrealistic expectations about what I can accomplish on any given day often leaves me frustrated and ungrateful. This problem is exacerbated when cancer-related ailments affect me physically or emotionally.

Rest. While oncologists regularly order patients to rest physically, there is little they can do to relieve internal anxieties apart from prescribing mood-altering drugs. The habit of Sabbath rest is an incredible antidote to this problem.[27] Rabbi Abraham Heschel describes it as a respite of "tranquility, serenity, peace and repose," "an armistice in man's cruel struggle for existence," "an experience of paradise."[28] As we humbly trust God in a posture of gratitude, we relax.

Our emotional health is directly tied to our ability to regularly detach from the demands of daily life. Sabbath rest encourages us to find a spiritual place that transcends physical space—to step away from the snowball effects of everyday living. Since my law school days, the Sabbath has been a consistent twenty-four-hour vacation. Even when work required 40 percent of my time on the road, I allocated a day to rest. Though the exact day of the week was flexible, the practice remained constant.

Things changed during my year-long recovery from MDS. Since I was unable to attend church with others, a new framework emerged. It included a longer prebreakfast time of Scripture reading, prayer, and two long walks. Mary and I watched our pastor online, and I followed a long-standing practice of taking a ninety-minute afternoon bath (often falling asleep). Once a week or so, I journaled about events, hopes, and fears.

Whatever your six-day pattern looks like, the seventh day is to be different. For those who no longer work, it is tempting to dismiss the Sabbath as now being irrelevant. Nothing could be further from the truth. It remains a special gift from God. Go to church, take a walk, converse with a faraway loved one, nap, read a book, or play a game.

Sabbath rest serves another purpose as well. It enables us to recognize that we are not indispensable to the world's well-being.

At times, we may fear that horrible things will happen if we get off the treadmill. Taking time away is the perfect cure for control over-reach. Inflating our sense of self is not only stressful, it is also counterproductive and ultimately self-destructive.

Rejecting illusion. As we humbly learn to trust, be grateful, and rest, we turn our backs on the illusion of control. Recognizing the foolishness of pushing buttons that aren't connected, we stop pretending that we control the future. By exercising appropriate control—neither too much nor too little—we enter into true freedom. Henri Nouwen summarizes: "Not clutching what we have . . . not trying to choreograph our own lives but surrendering to the God whom we love and want to follow. God invites us to experience our not being in control as an invitation to faith."[29]

REFLECTION QUESTIONS

1. Do you suffer from either control overreach or underreach? If so, describe a situation that you handled poorly.

2. Reviewing the four traits of appropriate control—humility, trust, gratitude, and rest—how do you self-assess your attitude and conduct?

3. Reflect on excerpts from the following three psalms. What lessons do you derive from them?

Psalm 3

Many are saying of me,
    "God will not deliver him."
But you, Lord, are a shield around me,
    my glory, the One who lifts my head high.

I call out to the LORD,
    and he answers me from his holy mountain.
I lie down and sleep;
    I wake again, because the LORD sustains me.
I will not fear though tens of thousands
    assail me on every side. (vv. 2-6)

Psalm 127

Unless the LORD builds the house,
    the builders labor in vain.
Unless the LORD watches over the city,
    the guards stand watch in vain.
In vain you rise early
    and stay up late,
toiling for food to eat—
    for he grants sleep to those he loves. (vv. 1-2)

Psalm 131

My heart is not proud, LORD,
    my eyes are not haughty;
I do not concern myself with great matters
    or things too wonderful for me.
But I have calmed and quieted myself,
    I am like a weaned child with its mother;
    like a weaned child I am content.
Israel, put your hope in the LORD
    both now and forevermore.

6

DEPENDING ON OTHERS

There are only four kinds of people in the world.
Those who have been caregivers.
Those who are currently caregivers.
Those who will be caregivers.
Those who will need a caregiver.

ROSALYNN CARTER

I take care of a parent with cancer. I sometimes take multiple
showers each day to hide the fact that I'm crying.

ANONYMOUS

Never doubt that a small group of thoughtful, committed individuals
can change the world: indeed, it's the only thing that ever has.

MARGARET MEAD

The friend who can be silent with us in a moment of despair or confusion,
who can stay with us in an hour of grief and bereavement, who can tolerate
not knowing, not healing, not curing . . . that is a friend who cares.

HENRI NOUWEN

ANCER UNDERCUTS OUR SENSE of self-sufficiency. Not only do we control less than we imagined, but our need for help from others is far greater. For a season, Mary had to do virtually everything on my behalf. I couldn't shower without assistance, stand in lines to pick up meds, or think clearly enough to organize my days.

For many of us, this vulnerability is a difficult transition. Moving from a position of perceived strength to a posture of dependence is humbling. After all, the myth of the rugged individual—independent and fearless—is deeply entrenched in Western culture.

In the early days of television, the series *Twilight Zone* ran an episode about an introverted bank teller named Henry. Hounded at work and henpecked at home, all Henry wants is to be left alone with his books. One day, while reading in the bank's vault during lunch, a nuclear bomb detonates. Exiting the vault, he discovers that he is the only survivor. As he walks about town, he finds a wing of the library still standing with enough books to last his remaining years. Smiling, he bends down to pick one up. But stumbling, his glasses fall off and are smashed. Without them, he is nearly blind and can't read. Realizing that no optometrist survived the blast, he is despondent.[1]

The moral of Henry's story? We need each other. As the seventeenth-century poet John Donne famously wrote: "No man is an island, entire of itself; every man is a piece of the continent, a part of the main."[2] Sociologist Brené Brown elaborates, "We pride ourselves on our independence and not depending on anyone. But social connection is one of our fundamental needs."[3]

By necessity, cancer patients are compelled to accept help. We don't cure ourselves; a community of caregivers does. When we pray the Lord's Prayer—"give us this day our daily bread"—we generally don't expect God to directly provide our sustenance. Rather, as Martin Luther observed, the Lord works through farmers, bakers, and grocers. They are the ones who sow, reap, bake, and sell.[4] In our context, God's good purposes are accomplished through doctors, nurses, pharmacists, and loved ones.

As survivors, we give tribute to a pantheon of heroes we depended on during treatment and recovery. Providing physical, emotional, and spiritual nurture, they fall into three broad groups: loved ones, medical professionals, and fellow cancer patients. Several of mine are cited on the dedication page of this book.

FAMILY AND FRIENDS

Family. Most of us have loved ones who have walked with us on our medical journeys—bearing disproportionate, unrecognized, and unpaid burdens. They are truly remarkable caregivers. While medical professionals are special, they do not go home with us. Only family members (or very close friends) care for us behind closed doors.

My brother Grant literally gave part of himself. My pastor, Chris, stubbornly insisted that I seek medical assistance. Laura, our eldest, helped on several diagnostic visits. Carolyn read books with me and provided counsel regarding PTSD. Hundreds prayed, including many I've never met. But, of all my caregivers, one gave more than the rest combined, my wife, Mary.

PROFILE: MARY

When we married in our midtwenties, could Mary have had any idea what she was getting into? Could she have possibly grasped what "for better or worse" might entail?

My first cancer was bad enough. She had to perform medical procedures that no spouse should ever have to do. (I'll spare you the details.) But the onus placed on her during the second cancer was simply over-the-top—both in intensity and duration.

Following my diagnosis with MDS, Mary handled insurance headaches, made appointments, monitored my meds, cooked special meals, played chauffeur, did innumerable loads of laundry, and continuously cleaned and disinfected our unit. She also single-handedly prepped and sold our Wisconsin condo, gave away most of our possessions, rented storage space in Madison and Seattle, and moved us into our new home.

Most significantly, she gave me hope, love, and stability when I was at my lowest. Daily, she posted something clever on our bathroom mirror to lift my spirit as we counted down the number of days until we could return home. An artist, her cartoons captured the pathos of our situation—simultaneously funny and somber.

The title "caregiver" simply fails to do her justice. She carried me. Mary was so good at her role that my oncologist suggested she hire herself out to other patients. While this was intended to be a compliment, she responded (without hesitation): "No thank you. Caring for Alec was more than enough!"

Like Mary, Lucy Kalanithi cared for her husband, Paul, when he was sick. Reflecting on their final year together, her words are reminiscent of Mary's loving care for me:

We were as inseparable as we had been as students, when we held hands during lectures. Now we held hands in his coat pocket during walks outside after chemotherapy, Paul in a winter coat and hat even when the weather turned warm. He knew he would never be alone, never suffer unnecessarily. At home in bed a few weeks before he died, I asked him, "Can you breathe okay with my head on your chest like this?" His answer: "It's the only way I know how to breathe."[5]

Friends. Volunteer caregivers come in all shapes and sizes. Eight friends of Joni Eareckson Tada, a quadriplegic, take turns rotating her in bed at night to prevent bedsores. Their kindness allows her husband, Ken—the primary caregiver—to sleep through the night.[6]

In Mark's Gospel we read of a paralytic who is unable to approach Jesus on his own. Four friends step up to carry him on a stretcher to the house where Jesus is teaching. Blocked by a crowd, they boldly climb on the roof, cut a hole in it, and lower their friend via ropes to the master's feet. What an amazing image of a caregiving community.[7] Undaunted, they overcome every obstacle and doggedly pursue his cure.

Research shows that strong family connections and friendships are critical to recovery. Those with such support have a 50 percent chance of increased longevity. Being loved is more life sustaining than avoiding obesity, smoking, or high blood pressure.[8] Dean Ornish, professor of medicine at the University of California, San Francisco, concludes,

> I am not aware of any other factor in medicine—not diet, not exercise, not stress, not genetics, not drugs, not surgery—that has a greater impact on our quality of life. . . .
>
> Anything that promotes a sense of love and intimacy, connection, and community is healing.[9]

PROFESSIONAL CAREGIVERS

While loved ones may feel *compelled* to care for us, helping *strangers* is an entirely different genre. Medical practitioners in the field of oncology make a conscious decision to serve the sick and dying. A grim calling, it is easy to understand why there's a shortage of nurses entering the specialty today.[10] Something extra is required to embrace those who are horribly sick, regularly crabby, and far-too-often terminal.

Lacking expertise and capacity, patients are highly dependent on professional caregivers: from the person who draws our blood to the lab technician who reads the results, from the pharmacist who dispenses drugs to the radiologist who targets our tumors, from the oncologist who crafts a medical strategy to the physician's assistant who administers care, from the receptionist who greets us to the scheduler who juggles incredible complexity.

I suspect that every cancer survivor has a list of memorable medical caregivers. They welcomed us, made us feel important as individuals (not just as patients to be served professionally), and touched us in our most helpless moments. In short, we relied on them. Our very lives were in their hands.

Dearest to my heart are the infusion nurses, aides, and staff on the fifth floor at the Seattle Cancer Care Alliance. Entering my life when I was in pain and fearful, for eighty-seven consecutive days they checked my vitals and hooked my chest catheter to bags of hanging liquids. The tediousness of being tethered for up to four hours a day was offset by their cheerfulness, professionalism, and—dare I say—love. They fluffed pillows under my feet, covered me with warm blankets, and even brought chocolate milk.[11]

Mary and I entered their world as sojourners but quickly felt fully embraced. They adopted us into their family and fought hard not to lose me. Often providing insider information that doctors didn't, they listened to our fears and gave us incredible comfort—both physical and emotional. I will honor them all by briefly mentioning two.

When Jan first entered my infusion room, it was a complete surprise. Hers was a familiar face. Mary and I had known her as a college student two decades earlier. She had been in our home often as part of a Bible study group that Mary coled. Now, with roles reversed, she served as my nurse. Her kindness and competency quickly put us at ease. It was so reassuring to be in the care of someone who provided a connection to the outside world.

Karen offered levity laced with plainspokenness. I'll never forget Halloween when she dressed as the infamous Nurse Ratched of *One Flew Over the Cuckoo's Nest*. Exactly my type of humor. Commuting to work, she prayed for each patient. We often discussed spiritual things. She once confided with a wink: "Here's a little secret—we have to kill you to save you." While this may sound ghoulish at face value, we found it to be a helpful explanation of the transplant process.[12]

Superb professional caregivers exhibit three qualities. First, they are deeply missional, displaying a profound sense of commitment to aid the sick (and to eradicate cancer). Recognizing their work as a noble calling, they endure a rollercoaster of emotional ups and downs.

Second, despite depressing circumstances, they bring hope to their patients. As Proverbs observes, "A cheerful look brings joy to the heart; good news makes for good health."[13] They convey good spirits—even humor—in places of deep pain and sadness. Perhaps I should not have been surprised by the number of nurses who were people of faith. But there sure were a lot of them. Balancing empathy and fortitude, they were able to remain hopeful and steadfast even in dire cases.

Third, professional caregivers are holistic, caring not only for physical needs but emotional ones as well. In the parable of the good Samaritan (as recounted by Luke, a doctor), Jesus lauds the caregiver who "took pity . . . bandaged his wounds, pouring on oil and wine. Then he . . . took care of him."[14] Excellent caregivers go far beyond taking our pulse or giving shots. They connect with us at a deeply personal level.

Ministering to the most vulnerable, medical professionals are able to go where clergy cannot. They operate in a unique sphere, touching our bodies with healing hands. In doing so, they leave a legacy in our souls. To this day, Pope Francis remains deeply grateful to a nurse who cared for him as a young man: "Nurses are experts in humanity," "promoters of life and dignity," and "truly irreplaceable"; "Like no other, they have direct and continuous relationship with patients, take care of them every day, listen to their needs, and contact their very body. . . . We must recognize the importance of the simple gesture of touch."[15]

I encourage you to thank God for each of your professional caregivers by name, praying for their well-being. It is one of my great joys to seek mine out and dispense hugs during oncology visits. From their spontaneous responses, it is apparent that my life means something special to them as well.

PROFILE: DAMIEN DE VEUSTER, MODEL CAREGIVER

Father Damien was a nineteenth-century Belgian priest who, fully understanding the risks, volunteered to serve at a leper colony in Hawaii. Once he entered the quarantined community, he knew that he could never leave. Stepping on to the island of Molokai was a one-way ticket, but Damian felt called by the Lord.

Beyond providing spiritual care for members of his parish, he also acted as de facto doctor for everyone on the island—lancing sores, treating ulcers, and dressing wounds.

Finding residents living in squalor, he lobbied the government for building supplies. Men (many with missing limbs) were recruited to haul lumber to a planned village site. As they labored on the construction project, their sense of self-worth grew. The new cottages and gardens—orderly and attractive—were well-built.

Eleven years after his arrival, Father Damien stood to deliver a sermon one Sunday: "My brethren, *we* lepers . . ." In attending to others so intimately, he had contracted their disease. Rather than rue his fate, he developed an even greater bond with them.

In his remaining four years of life (dying at age forty-nine), he continued to serve Molokai's residents. Though physically impaired, he superintended the building of several more structures, including an orphanage. As his body disintegrated, he identified even more with members of his community.

Today, Father Damien is widely recognized as a remarkable spiritual leader and exemplary caregiver.[a] He is honored worldwide as an extraordinary human being who gave his life for others.

[a] John Farrow, *Damien the Leper* (New York: Image Books, 1954).

FELLOW CANCER PATIENTS

Is there anything worse than suffering alone? When in pain, we crave to be with fellow travelers. The speed with which these emotional ties are built is incredible. That's why parents who lose a child join grief groups, alcoholics attend AA meetings, military veterans support each other, divorcees join small groups, refugees start mutual assistance associations, and cancer families form support circles.[16]

The physical isolation mandated by my treatment was particularly difficult. Wanting desperately to be with my tribe—other MDS patients—I cheated the rules every chance I got to trade information and exchange encouragement. I devised ways to talk with them in the blood-draw lobby, elevators, and waiting rooms. Suffering by oneself is simply too hard. Many patients, who are not physically housed with their peers, seek support through online groups.

After Jerry Sittser lost his wife, daughter, and mother in a fatal car crash, he had conflicting impulses—both to withdraw and to engage others: "Though loss is a solitary experience we must face alone, it is also a common experience that can lead us to community. It can create a community of brokenness. We must enter the darkness of loss alone, but once there we will find others with whom we can share life together."[17]

Suffering creates an unanticipated sense of belonging. Even now—post-treatment—I continue to pursue transplant patients. This includes serving as a volunteer mentor to many who are newly diagnosed. As a card-carrying member of a unique group, I feel compelled to give back. There is an indescribable bond of identity and suffering that binds us together.

In his Pulitzer Prize-winning book, *The Emperor of All Maladies: A Biography of Cancer*, Siddhartha Mukherjee shares the story of Barbara Bradford. In the early 1990s, she was leading a Seattle area Bible study when she felt an unusual bulge near her collarbone. Realizing that her breast cancer had spread, she believed she would die soon.

When Barbara joined a "hail Mary" nine-week clinical trial, she noted how depressed the other fourteen breast-cancer patients appeared. Since hers was the only visible tumor, the women started a weekly ritual of touching the lump on her collarbone before receiving their dosage of drugs. Comparable to a basketball team joining hands in a huddle, her grotesque growth oddly brought fellow sufferers together. As the tumor began to shrink—slowly at first and then rapidly—hopes soared. Decades later, Barbara is still alive and regularly makes herself available to cancer patients.[18]

Four decades ago, only twelve of one hundred patients in the first bone-marrow-transplant clinical trial survived for a year.[19] I am the beneficiary of all those heroic souls who made today's science possible. Though strangers to me, my survival is based on their sacrifice. In other words, my dependence invisibly extends far beyond those I can see.

CAREGIVER DIFFICULTIES

Thus far, my observations about caregivers have all been upbeat. Sadly, life is often more complicated.

Relationships between survivors and caregiving loved ones are like a poem in three stanzas—precancer, treatment, and post-treatment. In my case, the first and third phases are quite similar. Reestablishing equilibrium with Mary, though challenging at times, has been relatively simple. While I am extremely grateful that she bore 100 percent of the load during my treatment, I am equally thankful (as is she) that we have been able to move back to a roughly 50-50 balance in our relationship. Occasional medical surprises force us to adjust this calculus.

Even in normal times, relationships are fluid. But what happens if ongoing health problems create imbalance, making mutual dependence impossible? What if the post-treatment dynamic places 75 percent of the burden on the caregiver? Or more? What if the survivor falls into a pattern of irritation and anxiety? What if the caregiver becomes overprotective or, in the alternative, collapses under the weight of responsibility?

Several factors adversely affect caregivers' relationships with their loved ones. Anger is a common emotion of survivors, often grounded in frustration, pain, and disempowerment.[20] It is easy to lash out at those who are most available. Sadness is another typical reaction. About a quarter of survivors experience some level of depression.[21] Others become passive and indecisive. At the extreme, a few will fall into *dependent personality disorder,* a one-way over-reliance on the caregiver.[22]

PROFILE: COLLEEN WRIGHT

Colleen is an elementary schoolteacher in North Carolina. When her husband was diagnosed with throat cancer, his oncologist told them that treatment would only be a "bump in the road." All would return to normal soon. At forty-six, he was physically fit and positive about the medical journey ahead.

They regularly sat through (weekly) chemo and (daily) radiation sessions together. Treatment went as expected. But shortly thereafter, unanticipated problems began to occur. Unable to swallow or drink without a tube, he began to lose weight. Variations in his blood pressure caused lightheadedness and loss of balance. Anxiety and depression set in. Days would pass when he wouldn't leave his bed. Blinds closed, he withdrew from Colleen and their two teenage daughters. He refused counseling and further tests.

Three years later, family life is quite different. Finances are tight. Fewer friends drop by for visits. He has lost a great deal of weight and—due to a significant depletion of energy and loss of muscle mass—is unable to help much around the house.

As a caregiver, Colleen now carries a heavy and unexpected load. Her roles as income earner, parent, medical supporter, transporter, insurance expert, financial manager, and housekeeper have all greatly expanded. She is tired much of the time and struggles to adjust to the "new normal."[a]

[a]Jane Hill, "How Caregivers Adjust to Post-Cancer Life," *CureToday.com*, March 14, 2013, www.curetoday.com/publications/cure/2013/spring2013/how-caregivers -adjust-to-post-cancer-life.

Colleen Wright's story is not uncommon. What started as a "regular procedure" for a "simple" cancer morphed into something far more onerous. Early in her husband's treatments, she was fully energized. But as the hoped-for sprint turned into a marathon, things changed. Funds that once went toward vacations were shifted to cover medical expenses. "Recovery" was no longer the finish line but an elusive aspiration. Sadly, cancer doesn't follow a set path.[23]

As the reality of a reduced life sinks in, many caregivers feel overwhelmed and even trapped. Some of you may ask, *Why me?* Every aspect of your life has become vulnerable to decline. Fatigue sets in. Managing kids becomes more difficult. Work evaluations suffer.

Caregiver burnout is a very real threat. A cancer specialist compares caregiving to holding a glass of water with an extended arm. At first, no problem. But ten minutes later, an ache starts to set in. Within half an hour, it becomes impossible to maintain the posture.[24]

Many of you feel guilty even acknowledging your own needs. After all, you reason, "my suffering is minimal compared to that of my loved one." An alarming number of caregivers lapse into depression.[25] To remain emotionally healthy, professionals recommend seeking support from family members, friends, and social service agencies. One study shows that only 13 percent of caregivers receive regular respites.[26]

Sadly, some caregivers simply exit. While the divorce rate of married couples dealing with cancer is comparable to the general population, a huge gender gap exists. Whereas 97 percent of wives stay with husbands who have cancer, only 79 percent of husbands do likewise for their ailing wives.[27] As a male, I am embarrassed by this statistic. It is only slightly consoling that another study indicates that male caregivers who stay are more likely to regard their experience as positive than their female counterparts. The most stressed-out group of caregivers? Adult daughters.[28]

Abandoned survivors face a double hit—fighting cancer and being rejected by their mates. No wonder they use more antidepressants and are less likely to complete their treatments or participate in clinical trials.[29] Emotionally wounded, many lose hope and trust in others.

CAREGIVERS: PLEASE TAKE CARE OF YOURSELVES

Amid much turmoil, it is vital that you not neglect your own needs. Make time for daily prayer, Scripture reading, church attendance, and Sabbath rest. You may also find it helpful to talk with a pastor, see a licensed counselor, or join a support group. Regular exercise and being with friends are also important.

A researcher warns: "Caregivers are taking on a tremendous amount of responsibilities, almost like a second job, and they're apparently not taking very good care of themselves. They might be setting themselves up to be the next generation of care recipients."[30]

Cancer is a great disrupter, introducing dramatic shifts into many relationships. Reallocating responsibilities is highly taxing. The resultant stress leads many to seek outside assistance—both in terms of finding additional extra helping hands and identifying outside expertise. Adjusting to new realities can be complex, confusing, and challenging.

Above all, remember that you are not alone. God sees you. An embracing church is nearby. Others—both professionals and volunteers—can help you shoulder the load.

CAREGIVER RESOURCES

The American Cancer Society (ACS) provides remarkable resources for caregivers—including a 126-page guide, a caregiver hotline, and helpful videos. Topics include knowing your limits, juggling work and caregiving, dealing with new relational dynamics, communicating well, making medical decisions, pursuing respite care, and raising children. In addition, ACS can connect you to a support group of other caregivers, either virtually or face-to-face.[a]

[a]"Caregivers and Family," American Cancer Society, accessed May 2, 2019, www.cancer.org/treatment/caregivers.html.

REFLECTION QUESTIONS

1. Survivors:

- What lessons has cancer (or other suffering) taught you about being dependent on others?

- Name your caregivers. Pray for them. Thank God for their care.

2. Caregivers:

- What has been positive about your experience?

- What has been difficult?

- How well have you taken care of yourself?

3. Mutual dependence: reflect on 1 Corinthians 12:21-26:

> The eye cannot say to the hand, "I don't need you!" And the head cannot say to the feet, "I don't need you!" On the contrary, those parts of the body that seem to be weaker are indispensable, and the parts that we think are less honorable we treat with special honor. . . .

> But God has put the body together, giving greater honor to the parts that lacked it, so that there should be no division in the body, but that its parts should have equal concern for each other. If one part suffers, every part suffers with it; if one part is honored, every part rejoices with it.

4. Providing comfort: reflect on 2 Corinthians 1:3-7:

> Praise be to the God and Father of our Lord Jesus Christ, the Father of compassion and the God of all comfort, who comforts us in all our troubles, so that we can comfort those in any trouble with the comfort we ourselves receive from God. For just as we share abundantly in the sufferings of Christ, so also our comfort abounds through Christ. If we are distressed, it is for your comfort and salvation; if we are comforted, it is for your comfort, which produces in you patient endurance of the same sufferings we suffer. And our hope for you is firm, because we know that just as you share in our sufferings, so also you share in our comfort.

7

IDENTITY

Who Am I Now?

*To my friends I'm Ruth with cancer, not just
plain Ruth. Your identity does change.*
ANONYMOUS

*To me, survivorship is very much an attitude;
it's a state of mind. How we interpret the experience
of cancer and integrate it into our lives
is fundamental to how we coexist with it.*
SELMA SCHIMMEL

*An identity would seem to be arrived at by the way
in which the person faces and uses his experience.*
JAMES BALDWIN

*This brush with our own mortality offers cancer survivors
a good chance to figure out who we authentically are.*
BARBARA TAKO

C ANCER CHANGES US. Regardless of our age, gender, ethnicity, education, or economic status, each of us emerges with an altered sense of self. We are not only different physically but psychologically and socially as well.

While some modifications are obvious (e.g., loss of a body part), others are frustratingly obscure (e.g., forgetfulness). Scholars refer to these adjustments as "renegotiating identity," "validating the altered self," and "writing a new biography."[1] The question *who am I now?* may take years to sort out.

My story is unusual in that my treatment actually altered my genes. A swab taken from inside my cheek collects birth DNA, but blood drawn now carries the DNA of my brother Grant. Yes, the transplant changed my blood type. And, yes, I now have two distinct side-by-side sets of DNA. Scientists label transplant survivors like me *chimeras*, a word first used in Homer's *Iliad* to describe a hybrid monster with a lion's head, a goat's body, and a serpent's tail. Thankfully, the definition broadened over time to include mermaids, centaurs, and other beings with incongruent parts like me.[2]

So, how should I feel about being Frankenstein-esque? Thankful, of course. I'm alive. But it does present some rather odd identity questions. Post-transplant, our youngest daughter, Carolyn, cleverly inquired, "Are you now my dad or my uncle?"

Cancer is a watershed event that divides our lives between BC (before cancer) and AD (after diagnosis). If given a choice between our BC and AD selves—what we look like, how we feel, how we perceive others regard us—most of us would gladly select the former.

Mo Gawdat, a senior leader at Google, has developed a helpful concept: "the expectation gap." The gap describes the dissonance between hopes and reality in everyday life. Examples include home sellers ("I expected to receive a higher offer from the buyer"), employees ("my boss said one thing but did another"), and spouses ("what I got is not what he promised").

Cancer survivors experience a variety of expectation gaps. Remembering how our bodies used to function, we lament our current physical limitations, ongoing pains, and fear of recurrence. How well we navigate the gap between what we used to be and what we are now will determine the quality of our new lives.

My first cancer presented few identity problems. Able to pretty much return to my old self, I didn't struggle with gaps. However, such was certainly not the case with my second round. It forced me to renegotiate the question *Who am I now?* on many levels.

The question of identity provides a stark contrast between secular and biblical values. While Western culture focuses on temporal concerns such as appearance, career, and acceptance by others, followers of Jesus are grounded in an eternal perspective. This rooted sense of self allows us to approach cancer differently.

We will now explore three aspects of identity—self-perception, our bodies, and our social roles.

OUR SELF-PERCEPTION

How we view ourselves vis-à-vis cancer is critical to our sense of identity. In a recent survey, a post-treatment group of eighteen-to-fifty-five-year-olds were asked to describe themselves as either "victims," "patients," or "survivors." The results are revealing. Those who self-identified as "victims" experienced lower life satisfaction, feelings of powerlessness, and abused alcohol and drugs at a much higher rate than the other two categories. At the other end of the spectrum, those who saw themselves as "survivors" experienced greater self-esteem, better mental health, and a renewed sense of purpose.[3]

When we are first diagnosed, it is natural to feel like victims. That's why our initial reaction is often *why me?* However, if we allow ourselves to linger too long in this space, we become mired in a pit of hopelessness, bitterness, and entitlement. Putting on a cloak of injustice, we begin to blame others for our situation. Psychologists label this behavior as taking on "the sick person role." Expecting others to meet our needs ad infinitum creates a downward cycle of despair and isolation.[4]

Similarly, if we hold on to the title of "patient" too long—even after we are safely on the road to recovery—our journey to wellness is delayed. As we regain agency, exercising appropriate control becomes important lest we lapse back into victimhood. For most of us, a time comes when it is right to self-identify as a "survivor." Having said that, it is important to acknowledge that some patients are simply unable to make this move. Chronic maladies or new health problems impede their progress.

My second cancer reflects all three stages. When my life hung in the balance, I was a "deathly sick man." Then, as good medical news began to filter in, I transitioned to a "fragile patient." Finally, about two years later, I gained sufficient confidence to call myself a "survivor." These transitions are not always easy. A colon cancer survivor says, "Using the term 'survivor' to describe myself was one of the hardest things I had to overcome. I was superstitious about it and afraid to use it. It took me years to feel comfortable saying (in the past tense), 'I had cancer.'"[5]

In due course, if we are fortunate, we progress along this continuum. Though the road can be bumpy, God provides various graces along the way. These include a strong sense of his presence as well as the support of loved ones and caring professionals. As we heal, cancer moves off the front burner and no longer dominates our thoughts multiple times a day.[6] We begin to not only survive but to survive well.

PROFILE: SABRINA GAUER

After graduating from college, Sabrina recorded a music album and did some touring. Eventually, she landed a job as a church worship leader. Life was good. She looked forward to meeting someone special, getting married, and having kids.

Then she was diagnosed with stage 4 oral cancer, quite a blow for a rising singer. During a six-hour surgery, half her tongue was removed and reconstructed with muscle from her neck and left arm. "I felt as if the rug had been yanked out from beneath my 27 year old sense of identity."

Looking back, Sabrina reflects, "I am a completely different person now. Something amazing is growing and shaping inside me. Cancer has given me a deeper perspective—not based on what others think, or the shallow sense of success and identity. I'm continuing to become who I was created to be."

While she struggles with bodily limitations, such as a dysfunctional shoulder and daily soreness in her neck, she observes: "While cancer will always be a part of my story, and the nightmarish year my body betrayed me is literally carved into my arm, neck, and tongue, my identity is not based on ever-changing circumstances. First and foremost, my life belongs to Jesus."[a]

[a]Sabrina Gauer, "Finding My Identity After Cancer," *First Descents*, accessed May 3, 2019, https://firstdescents.org/identity-battling-cancer.

Sabrina inspires us to root our identities in something secure and long-lasting. However fragile our "jars of clay" may be, we are first and foremost children of God. We exist in a story much larger than ourselves and a faith community that extends far beyond what we can see. Our sense of self isn't based on things that are here today and gone tomorrow, but on our relationship with a loving heavenly Father.[7]

OUR BODIES

Adjusting to our altered bodies can be traumatic, especially if the gap between our expectations and reality is wide. Breast cancer survivors must deal with the aftermath of mastectomies. Testicular cancer patients have to regroup after surgical removal. Patients receiving hormonal therapy face a variety of side effects. Younger patients confront the horrible prospect of infertility—a seismic shift in identity.[8]

During a recent doctor's visit, I crossed paths with a man struggling to wheel himself to an appointment. I stopped, introduced myself, and asked if I could push him. Rick smiled appreciatively and said yes. It was apparent that his newly bandaged leg had been recently amputated and that he was uncomfortable using his wheelchair. As I took him to his doctor's office and turned from his warm goodbye, a tear ran down my cheek. I felt so sad for him. His situation was simply awful. As he recalibrates his identity and adjusts expectations, I pray that he will be able—in time—to make the transition from victim to survivor.

While nowhere as dramatic as Rick's condition, I have also had to acclimate to my new body. Donnell Thomas, the father of bone-marrow transplants, graphically described his cure, "We have to

burn down the house to kill the rats."[9] In other words, to save patients' lives, it is necessary to give massive doses of chemo, full body
radiation, and steroids. While extremely grateful to be alive, I am
fully aware that the torched house Dr. Thomas referred to is my body.

My oncologist says that treatments have "scrambled my cells."
This makes me more susceptible to a variety of secondary cancers.
Foremost on the list is skin cancer. Every morning, a three-inch
scar on my chest stares back at me in the bathroom mirror. A nearly
identical twin is on my back. While I've never regarded my torso
as being model-like, at times I feel like a Raggedy Andy doll. No
doubt, more melanoma-related surgeries will follow. Even on rainy
Seattle days, I must wear liberal doses of sunscreen, long-sleeved
shirts, long pants, and a nerdy broad-rimmed hat.

Likewise, since full body radiation "fried my cartilage" (as another specialist put it), arthritis is also part of my new reality. As a
person who has always prided himself as being physically fit, it is
sometimes painful just to put my socks on. My reaction to these
changes? A mixture of frustration, grief, and (at times) embarrassment. I hate limping in public.

But, lest I whine, others face far more serious body identity
issues. I have an InterVarsity colleague who lost his entire arm,
shoulder and all, to cancer. Another friend has non-Hodgkin's lymphoma, a cancer that—though beaten back and dormant for years
at a time—never goes away. Nearly three years ago, he contracted
shingles. Lodged in the sinus cavity of his forehead, it produces
constant—sometimes debilitating—headaches.

What is remarkable about these two men is that, despite dramatic changes to their bodies, each has adjusted to a new normal.
One continues to minster to college students while the other has

become (in my opinion) the world's best grandfather. Somehow, they have been able to narrow the expectation gap, inspiring me to face my own limitations and be more thankful for my extended life. I also take solace in the fact that Scripture promises a fully restored resurrected body in heaven.[10] I look forward to running again.

Sexuality. Cancer can also adversely impact our ability to be active sexual partners. Some survivors are no longer able to perform physically. Others lose their desire for sex due to feeling less attractive. About half of women with reproductive organ and breast cancers report long-term sexual dysfunction. The same is true for men receiving prostate treatment.[11]

Assessing my masculinity over the past eight years has been a difficult part of my identity journey. Prior to cancer, sex was a meaningful and enjoyable part of my relationship with Mary. Without going into great detail, surgery to address my first cancer greatly reduced my libido. But it was the treatment for my second cancer that made me impotent. I confess that writing this is uncomfortable.

So who am I now in terms of my male identity? I share my story because it is common not just for men with reproductive cancers but for all who receive harsh treatments. Compared to saving my life, this side effect is a small price to pay. However, there are times that I feel a deep sense of loss and even (irrational) shame.

Many women experience a similar challenge to their femininity. In a study of mastectomy patients, participants spoke in stark terms about their altered identities. Comments include:

Half of me is missing. . . . I don't want to look in the mirror. . . .
I was beautiful but now I feel ugly. . . . I am ashamed. . . . I am

incomplete. . . . I can't use my right arm due to the removal of lymph nodes. . . . I don't want to show myself to my husband.[12]

Postmastectomy, many women expect to return to a proximity of their former selves via reconstructive surgery. But it is an imperfect science, often leading to significant disappointment. If one's postcancer body doesn't approximate its precancer version, a second wave of grief and embarrassment can hit.[13]

The impact on our partners can also be dramatic. When couples are unable to engage sexually, their loss extends far beyond the physical realm. Some of the sweetest moments in human relationships exist in the context of sexual activity.

My journey to a new definition of masculinity has not been easy. Redefining who I am took the better part of a year. I spent a fair amount of time lamenting to God and having long talks with Mary. Gradually, I recalibrated expectations and moved into a better place. Though sexually inactive, I am still very much a man.

Mary and I have found other ways to be intimate. Our love is deep and joyful. If anything, this is the sweetest season of our marriage. Though certainly more difficult for younger couples, it is possible for relationships to successfully navigate cancer-altered bodies. Inviting a counselor into the conversation may ease the transition.

OUR SOCIAL ROLES

Personal identity is also tied up in our social roles. Think of the questions strangers ask each other when they first meet: "What do you do?" "Where are you from?" "How large is your family?" We self-define by our clans, our jobs, our hometowns, our competencies, and our future aspirations. When cancer interrupts any of these anchor identities, our sense of who we are is jolted, sometimes severely.[14]

My social roles include husband, father, brother, uncle, employee, friend, neighbor, and parishioner. Thus, it came as a shock when—in a period of just three weeks after diagnosis—I stepped down from my InterVarsity leadership position, left a Wisconsin community (and church) we dearly loved, and moved two thousand miles for treatment. Life turned on a dime. The abrupt shift from high-touch leader to isolated patient profoundly tested my sense of self.

Family members and friends. Though I felt total support from loved ones, other survivors are not so fortunate. Sadly, it is all too common for friends and family members to disengage during treatment. PJ Hamel watched as her best friend went AWOL just as she was most vulnerable. Advising other survivors, she writes,

> It's not you that's causing this sudden rewiring of the relationship network—it's your disease. Your friends are giving you a rare inner glimpse of themselves. Who's strong, capable, and optimistic? Who's inwardly terrified about health issues? Who, as a young child, witnessed a grandmother's painful death from breast cancer and simply can't chance going there again?[15]

Years later, PJ reconnected with her friend. When the latter was asked why she had disappeared, she sheepishly replied, "I was scared. Scared of cancer. Scared you would die. And I wasn't strong enough to face down those fears, so I walked away."[16]

PROFILE: BRIAN AND LORRAINE KEMBER

An outgoing Australian couple, Brian and Lorraine enjoyed a wide circle of friends. Welcomed in many homes, they also socialized extensively at a local club. However, things changed quickly after Brian was diagnosed with a rare cancer caused by asbestos fibers. Lorraine noticed that "people began to treat us differently." Instead of being embraced as she had hoped, many backed away.

This came as a real shock to her: "Cancer had entered our lives, but we were still Lorraine and Brian, and we needed our friends more than ever. Instead, we were greeted with silence, whispers, or attempts at joviality. No one, it seemed, could look us in the eye, nor could they remain in our company for long." Many detached rather than deal directly with Brian's situation.

"It seemed as if we had suddenly lost our identity and this hurt us both deeply." In time, some friends visited to inquire about Brian's cancer, but were visibly uncomfortable. These reactions hurt the Kembers anew, making them question whether the people they thought they knew well had ever really been friends at all. Eventually, a handful of people worked through the awkwardness and connected in a deeper way.[a]

[a]Lorraine Kember, "Why Friends Act the Way They Do After a Cancer Diagnosis," *Asbestos.com,* June 7, 2013, www.asbestos.com/blog/2013/06/07/why-friends-act-the-way-they-do-after-a-cancer-diagnosis.

PJ's and Lorraine's accounts are all too common. But they raise a haunting question: How many of us have disappeared when friends have gone through a divorce, lost a spouse, or become ill? Such self-reflection hopefully makes us less judgmental of others. As survivors, it behooves us to show grace to those who have disappointed us. Having experienced what it is like to be left behind, let us commit to never treating anyone else in a similar manner.

Social stigma can be particularly acute for those with specific cancers. Lung cancer survivors, for example, describe feeling ostracized by friends and coworkers. Since most people associate the illness with smoking (even though many patients have never lit up), shame and social isolation often result.[17] Likewise, those suffering from cirrhosis of the liver report experiencing intense stigmatization even though most of them are not heavy drinkers.[18]

This sense of rejection is exacerbated in some parts of the world where cancer is wrongly believed to be hereditary. This makes it difficult for young adults with sick parents to find spouses. Some cultures even associate cancer with evil spirits.[19]

Work. Many of us are guilty of intertwining our identities too tightly with our careers. By doing so, we risk defining ourselves not by whose we are but by what we do. This is particularly hazardous for overachievers like me. I deemed my work to be so important that I delayed being diagnosed for both cancers. Not wanting to lose my status, I foolishly jeopardized my health. Tim Keller warns that "elevating a good thing into an ultimate thing" constitutes idolatry.[20]

When cancer strikes, our roles as experts, leaders, problem solvers, and teammates are all at risk.

Thankfully, most survivors are not compelled to change jobs. After a season of recovery—perhaps including a period of disability—old positions are reassumed. Most supervisors and colleagues welcome us back. This was certainly my experience after I returned to work with InterVarsity post-transplant (albeit in a new role).

Sometimes, however, reentry is not a happy story. A major study of one thousand breast-cancer survivors found a 30 percent drop in employment over a four-year period. Why? While some women were physically unable to perform at the same level, the majority were willing and able. Reviewing the study, oncologist Elaine Schattner identifies several forms of subtle discrimination. When survivors miss work for doctors' appointments, display higher levels of fatigue, or are less able to travel, they are often passed over for plum assignments and promotions. Many are later demoted or released. Hitting a "cancer ceiling" is the regrettable experience of many survivors.[21]

OUR SPIRITUAL IDENTITY

Though scarred, slowed, and sometimes stigmatized, the core of who we are remains constant. Even on dark days, cancer cannot erase our spiritual identity. My friend Steve Hayner put it beautifully a few months before his death: "I remind myself that my primary identity is not as a cancer patient, but rather as a beloved child of God."[22]

Our heavenly Father knows who we are more intimately than anyone else. He weeps when we suffer and rejoices when we thrive. Our spiritual identities begin and end in him. Remarkably, he regards each of us as "his masterpiece." His goal is to transform us into his image.[23]

How can we fully appropriate this identity? By allowing him to work on our souls. By releasing our old normal. By leaning into an eternal perspective. By not focusing on temporal things. By redefining hope.

In a poem titled *Who Am I?* written shortly before his execution by the Nazis, Dietrich Bonhoeffer wrote, "Whoever I am, you know me, I am yours, O God."[24] Who are we now? We are daughters and sons of God being changed into his image. Though life may be challenging, we find strength in his presence and promises.

We are his beloved. This is our true identity.

REFLECTION QUESTIONS

1. Have you experienced an expectation gap between your before-cancer (BC) and after-diagnosis (AD) self? If so, describe. How have you handled the changes?

2. More specifically, have you struggled with identity issues related to (1) self-perception, (2) body image, or (3) social roles? What has helped you move forward?

3. Reflect on 1 John 3:1-3 and 2 Corinthians 4:7-10. What do these passages say to you?

See what great love the Father has lavished on us, that we should be called children of God! And that is what we are! . . . We know that when Christ appears, we shall be like him, for we shall see him as he is. All who have this hope in him purify themselves, just as he is pure.

We have this treasure in jars of clay, to show that this all-surpassing power is from God and not from us. We are hard pressed on every side, but not crushed; perplexed, but not in despair; . . . struck down, but not destroyed. We always carry around in our body the death of Jesus, so that the life of Jesus may also be revealed in our body.

PART THREE

LIVING IN BONUS TIME

LIVING LIKE LAZARUS

Earlier, soccer was presented as a metaphor for surviving cancer. Players run hard during *regulation time* and then a referee extends the game with supplementary minutes. This extra session—*bonus time*—symbolizes months, years, or even decades added to our lives. While none of us know how long this season will last, we are motivated to make the most of it. Acknowledging our unique opportunity, we reflect on what our lives might become.

Scripture tells of nine people who were granted bonus time.[1] The best known was Lazarus. A close friend of Jesus, he contracted a fatal illness and died. After he had lain in a tomb for four days, Jesus brought him back to life. Three weeks later, despite a "dead or alive" bounty being placed on Jesus' head by religious leaders, Lazarus boldly invited his healer to a celebratory dinner at his home. So visible was Lazarus's identification with Jesus that a decision was made to kill them both.[2]

When Jesus departed for Passion Week the next day, biblical references to Lazarus cease. What became of him? Greek Orthodox tradition says that Lazarus was thirty years old when he died the first time. Shortly thereafter, he fled persecution by moving to the island of Cyprus. There, he lived out his devotion to Jesus as a priest for another three decades before dying a second time at the age of sixty. It is easy to imagine that the direction of his bonus time (ages 31-60) differed significantly from his prior life.[3]

As cancer survivors, we (like Lazarus) have the opportunity to assess life anew and to reset direction. The next four chapters discuss how to make the most of bonus time by experiencing survivor's growth (chap. 8), clarifying purpose (chap. 9), using time well (chap. 10), and cultivating wonder (chap. 11).

8

SURVIVOR'S GROWTH

We can sink under the weight of adversity or
we can rise up to live better than before.
LYNN UNDERWOOD

Cancer is a spiritual practice that teaches me about faith and resilience.
KRIS CARR

I know God will not give me anything I can't handle.
I just wish that he didn't trust me so much.
MOTHER TERESA

The most beautiful people we know are those who have
known defeat,
known suffering,
known struggle,
known loss,
and have found their way out of the depths.
ELISABETH KÜBLER-ROSS

O VER THE PAST FEW YEARS, I've shared my medical story with several audiences. I'll never forget a questioner who—repeating one of my comments about becoming a better person—asked whether I was thankful for the cancer. Inside my head, I screamed, *Are you nuts? I wouldn't wish this experience on Hitler!* In my verbal response, however, I diplomatically stated that I hadn't blithely jumped between lightning bolts. I got hit. No thank you, I would not choose to do it again.

But the reality is that I've grown on my cancer journey. Though fully aware of my physical blemishes, I am more emotionally vibrant. A new level of toughness, hopefully informed by humility and a heart of wisdom, has emerged. Less bothered by trivial matters, I am—for the most part—happier.

That's what makes this chapter so challenging to write. What is the proper balance between acknowledging the horror of the journey while at the same time recognizing how much I've matured?

THE HOPE OF SURVIVOR'S GROWTH

In interviews with thousands of trauma survivors, psychologists Richard Tedeschi and James Calhoun of the University of North Carolina discovered that most patients move beyond recovery. Their balloons not only refill but actually expand over time, taking them to a higher level of life. This phenomenon is called *post-traumatic growth.*[1]

I will use a simpler term—*survivor's growth.* About a third of survivors experience it profoundly, a third mildly, and a third not at all (or even regress).[2] While our wounds, recurring pain, and physical limitations remind us of the gauntlet we've been through, there is also—for most us—a surprisingly positive side of the ledger. As crazy as it may sound, cancer can be a catalyst for personal development. "Productive suffering," as one scholar describes it, can transform us for good.[3]

Survivor's growth doesn't take us back to our precancer selves (point A). Neither do we get stuck at being cancer's victims (point B). Rather, as we adapt, it takes us to a new place where we've never been before (point C). We morph into different people. While much of our former selves carries forward, we are enhanced. Our beliefs and character are stretched, our worldviews challenged, and our resolve strengthened. Job, who certainly knew a great deal about such matters, observed, "The righteous keep moving forward, and those with clean hands become stronger and stronger."[4]

Unlike the day-to-day routine of our precancer lives, we have experienced profound disruption. This break from the status quo provides a unique opportunity for self-examination. What do we like about ourselves? What do we want to discard? Tedeschi and Calhoun label this process *rumination*. They advise, "The challenge is to see the opportunity presented by this earthquake. Don't just rebuild the same crappy building you had before. Why not build something better?"[5]

The concept that suffering—if rightly processed—can enhance personal growth strikes a deep biblical chord. In Scripture, pain is often regarded as a pathway to wisdom and holiness. God takes our brokenness, redeems it, and creates new life. The apostle James counsels: "Consider it pure joy, my brothers and sisters, whenever you face trials of many kinds, because you know that the testing of your faith produces perseverance. Let perseverance finish its work so that you may be mature and complete, not lacking anything."[6]

It is important to acknowledge, however, that some cancer patients do not bounce back. Sadly, the cumulative impact of so many negative changes can be overwhelming, leading to depression, anger, or even addiction. Factors such as fear of recurrence, ongoing pain levels, and pessimistic temperament appear to also play a role. In the Old Testament, King Hezekiah embodied such regression. When he contracted a deadly illness, he prayed and the Lord added fifteen years of bonus time. But then he dove into an emotional tailspin and ended poorly. Personal decline is a very real possibility.[7]

But for the two-thirds of us who experience survivor's growth, a variety of positive attributes often emerge. Tedeschi and Calhoun list several possible changes.[8] Roughly following their findings, we will focus on three—grit, spirituality, and boldness.

Grit. Author Angela Duckworth defines *grit* as tenacity, perseverance, passion, resilience, and toughness.[9] Through extended periods of suffering and insecurity, most cancer patients unconsciously nurture grit. While I wish the route to this virtue were easier, the fact remains that remarkable inner strength often develops. Although there can be no adequate payback for surgeries, chemo, and befuddling uncertainty we endure, grit is an undeniable byproduct of such circumstances.

Cancer forces us to adapt. In a landmark book about four hundred famous persons, Victor Goertzel found that 75 percent of them came from dysfunctional homes. Apparently, early childhood difficulties had a "steeling effect" that led to extraordinary personal strength.[10]

I suspect that we can all quickly name someone who developed great resilience despite facing many obstacles. My mom, the youngest of six kids, was only ten years old when the family farm was lost. Then her father abandoned the family. At age twenty-one, she joined the US State Department. Just two years later, she was promoted to report directly to the American ambassador in Spain. As the only sibling to finish college, she went on to graduate school and became the head of a large foreign-language department in the Seattle public schools. A single mom raising three sons, she personifies grit to me.

Jim Rendon tells a moving story about his father, a Holocaust survivor, in *Upside: The New Science of Post-Traumatic Growth*. Serving in the merchant marines, he was able to allay shipmates' fears about hauling seven tons of explosives across the Pacific Ocean. Notes Rendon: "My father calmed them down. It's not that he wasn't afraid, but that he'd already been through so much worse. His perspective was different."[11]

In his letter to the Romans, the apostle Paul provides a parallel teaching that adversity produces perseverance (or resilience). Such endurance nurtures a mature character that leads to greater hope.[12] The Greek word for character is *dokimē*, a military term used for a grizzled veteran (as opposed to a raw recruit). Paul praises the disciple who has been tested and passed.[13] In other words, if we allow him, God can repurpose our pain to make us better people.

Please note that grit must never be confused with the *power of positive thinking*. Some, like testicular cancer survivor Lance Armstrong, cite their indomitable willpower for their recovery. Armstrong credits his arduous work ethic, disciplined diet, and incredible energy for "winning" the cancer battle.[14] This is the same snake oil that Steve Jobs espoused.

Cancer is much too dominant an enemy for us to defeat on our own. We don't prevail over cancer. God does. Medical professionals do. Intercessors do. We are not agents of our healing, but recipients.

I recall proudly asking my oncologist whether being a physically fit nonsmoker had improved my chances of a successful transplant. His response slapped me down: "Not one bit." Bonus time should be approached with humility, not pride.

That said, grit does require us to diligently do our part. Employing *appropriate control* includes doggedly complying with doctors' orders, watching what we consume, getting enough sleep, and being consistent with our exercise routines. Research shows that staying physically fit has a significant long-term positive impact.[15]

PROFILE: MAARTEN VAN DER WEIJDEN

At nineteen, Maarten was a Dutch long-distance swimming champion. But in 2001 he was diagnosed with leukemia. His odds of surviving a bone-marrow transplant were 30 percent. For two years he lost complete control of his life, depending wholly on oncologists to shepherd him through massive doses of chemotherapy.

Three years later, he reentered the water cancer free. Setting modest goals at first, he swam in local competitions. Over the next five years, his strength gradually increased, as did his speed. At the 2008 Olympics in Beijing, he surprised everyone by winning the gold medal in the 10,000-meter marathon.

In a subsequent interview, he criticized Lance Armstrong's advocacy of positive thinking: "I think it's dangerous." Maarten knew that his life had not been saved by personal willpower but by forces outside himself. "I had 0% influence on surviving." Of course, using the grit developed during those difficult years caused him to train harder and smarter.

Taking advantage of bonus time, Maarten has seized every opportunity. After a successful career as a finance manager, he has set up a cancer foundation and is flourishing as an author, playwright, actor, entrepreneur, and motivational speaker. At thirty-seven, he is married and has two young daughters. Maarten embodies the essence of survivor's growth. His TED talk is incredibly inspiring.[a]

[a]David Feldman and Lee Kravetz, *Supersurvivors: The Surprising Link Between Suffering and Success* (New York: HarperCollins, 2014), 17-19.

Spirituality. Earlier, I reflected on the vibrancy of God's presence on my darkest days. I am thankful that I continue to enjoy his closeness. Strange to say, cancer has been a remarkable stimulant to my spiritual life. I pray longer, read Scripture more reflectively, express gratitude with greater regularity, and see divine wonder more frequently.

Still, I was surprised to discover that secular scholars regard my experience as normative rather than exceptional. Tedeschi and Calhoun, for example, use "spiritual change" as one of their five factors for patients who thrive post-trauma (attributes include "stronger religious faith" and "better understanding of spiritual matters"). While they don't precisely define faith—vaguely labeling it "existential"—the evidence is indisputable. There is no denying that sincere religious faith plays a significant role in *survivor's growth.*[16]

I was further taken aback to find more than 100 studies by scholars at prestigious institutions that affirm these findings.[17] As a group, survivors like me—who encounter God's personal touch on a daily basis—are much more likely to emerge from trauma with an increased sense of meaning, life satisfaction, self-esteem, harmony, and emotional well-being.[18] One report concludes, "Participants viewed surrender (to God) as . . . giving them an increased sense of overall purpose and meaning to their lives in their post-cancer experience."[19] A researcher at Fordham University concurs:

"Mature faith is a more powerful predictor of growth than personality or social support.... People who had secure relationships with God were moving through the grief and loss differently than those who had troubling relationships with God or were feeling abandoned by God."[20]

A study done at Yale four decades ago is particularly eye-opening. A group of Vietnam War pilots held as prisoners of war were interviewed postrelease. Despite horrific conditions, often resulting in severe physical pain (and later PTSD), 61 percent reported that they had actually benefitted from their captivity. Many pointed to a more robust religious faith. Contrary to expectations, those who suffered the harshest treatment recorded the most positive change. In a follow-up study conducted twenty-five years later, the results remained constant.[21]

Boldness. A third common attribute of survivor's growth is enhanced boldness. One researcher observes, "They are more adventurous, open to try new things, imaginative, and curious."[22] Caring less about failure and shame, survivors are liberated to act courageously, be authentic, and take more risks.

Boldness includes saying what we think. With less patience for banal small talk, fewer euphemisms and generalities are utilized. Cutting directly to the chase, most of us are now more candid.[23] We also feel more confident to pursue our sense of calling. Pam Parker, a survivor who struggles with depression, describes how cancer aids her as an author:

Cancer changed my attitude about my writing. Before, I was afraid to submit my work. I created stories but couldn't muster the courage to put them out in the world. I was afraid of rejection. Cancer slapped me in the face—you were afraid of a rejection letter from an editor?! Fear something worth fearing![24]

Some survivors have the audacity to step even further outside their comfort zones. My nominee for patron saint of boldness is a sixty-six-year-old Floridian named Helen Dunsford, with stage 4 cancer. Standing in line at a bank, a thirty-two-year-old robber suddenly appeared with a gun and demanded $10,000 from the teller. While everyone else complied with an order to lie flat on the floor, Helen ran, jumped, and bear-hugged the thief to the ground. As they tumbled, she yelled: "I've got cancer. You can kill me if you want." When police arrived, they were amazed to see Helen atop the suspect. Asked why she had risked her life, she responded, "I've got nothing to lose."[25]

While we may be hesitant to embrace Helen's radical approach, *appropriate boldness* is lauded throughout Scripture. When Joshua leads his people into the Promised Land, the Lord encourages him to "be strong and courageous." In Jesus' parable about ten talents, the daring man is commended and his faint-hearted peer condemned. Paul, who faced death several times, remained "very bold" even exhorting his lieutenant, Timothy, not to be "timid" but to operate out of "power."[26]

PROFILE: LEE RHODES

At thirty-two, Lee was a stay-at-home mom. While engaged in an annual physical exam, her three preschoolers colored in the waiting room. After a technician took x-rays, it struck her as odd that he avoided making eye contact with her. A doctor later told her that she had bronchial carcinoma, a rare form of lung cancer.

While enduring rounds of chemotherapy, she observed many of her peers missing treatments. She discovered that they couldn't afford to take time off from work, pay for child care, or cover downtown parking. This broke her heart. She was also touched when her husband brought her a cup he had made at a glass-blowing class. Lee placed a candle inside and found the glow extremely calming.

After recovering from cancer three years later, Lee hired a professional glassmaker and named her small company Glassybaby. Vowing to give 10 percent of revenues to assist poor cancer patients, she started selling the candleholders at street fairs and out of her garage.

Her boldness paid off. Fast forward two decades. After all the joys and failures of a start-up, Glassybaby has succeeded wildly. Today, it is a $20 million-dollar business with 338 staff and eight stores. Lee pays a living wage and provides health care for her employees. Over the past decade, her company has donated $8 million to four hundred charities serving cancer patients, and she has been honored as "entrepreneur of the year" by *Entrepreneur* magazine.

Lee's cancer reshuffled her life's cards, giving her a renewed sense of purpose, missional use of time, and extraordinary courage. Without cancer, she doubts that she would have discovered these things.[a]

[a]Susan Adams, "With Help from Jeff Bezos and Martha Stewart, a Cancer Survivor Turns Glassybaby into a $20m Company," *Forbes*, December 6, 2016, www.forbes.com/sites/forbestreptalks/2016/12/06/with-help-from-jeff-bezos-and-martha-stewart-a-cancer-survivor-turns-glassybaby-into-a-20m-company/#186a5da1334b.

COMPOST FOR GROWTH

Though cancer is horrible, it may—by the grace of God—be transformed into something productive. Many survivors not only experience resilience but actually grow through the ordeal. Learning to accept the "new me" is often a tortuous process, but once done it allows us to become grittier, more spiritual, and bolder.

Jerry Sittser handles the tension masterfully: "I didn't go through pain and come out the other side. Instead, I lived in it and found within that pain the grace to survive and eventually grow ... I absorbed the loss into my life, like soil receives decaying matter, until it became a part of who I am."[27]

Sittser's imagery of each of us being an ecosystem that uses every experience—including the rotten parts—is prescient. Our souls are like enriched soil, full of both decay and nutrition. Though counterintuitive, flourishing plants emerge from manure. *Survivor's growth* finds its foothold in the compost of pain.

REFLECTION QUESTIONS

1. Have you experienced or observed survivor's growth? If so, describe.

2. In what ways has your cancer (or that of your loved one) affected your spirituality?

3. Is anything holding you back from being bolder? What steps can you take to move forward?

4. Reflect on Psalm 27:1-6

> The LORD is my light and my salvation—
> whom shall I fear?
> The LORD is the stronghold of my life—
> of whom shall I be afraid?
> When the wicked advance against me
> to devour me,
> it is my enemies and my foes
> who will stumble and fall.

Though an army besiege me,
   my heart will not fear;
though war break out against me,
   even then I will be confident.
One thing I ask from the Lord,
   this only do I seek:
that I may dwell in the house of the Lord
   all the days of my life,
to gaze on the beauty of the Lord
   and to seek him in his temple.
For in the day of trouble
   he will keep me safe in his dwelling;
he will hide me in the shelter of his sacred tent
   and set me high upon a rock.
Then my head will be exalted
   above the enemies who surround me;
at his sacred tent I will sacrifice with shouts of joy.

9

CLARITY OF PURPOSE

Cancer can shuffle our values like a deck of cards.
SULEIKA JAOUAD

Suffering is wonderfully clarifying. It forces us
to ask basic questions about what is most important in life.
That's why many who suffer . . . become different people.
JERRY SITTSER

He who has a why to live for can bear almost any how.
VICTOR FRANKL

It took a life-threatening disease for me
to slow down and get the clarity I needed.
MICHAEL, TESTICULAR CANCER SURVIVOR

S URVIVING CANCER is a reset button.

Entering *bonus time* provides an extraordinary opportunity to redirect our lives. To focus on what's truly important. To deepen our relationship with God. To live more simply. To heal broken relationships. In short, to become better versions of ourselves.

Only one in four Americans claims a clear sense of purpose. In contrast, three out of four cancer survivors report having new goals, altered priorities, and a different outlook on life.[1] Why the disparity? Rabbi Yael Ridberg, a breast cancer survivor, reflects, "We don't usually take the opportunity to do this kind of deep work until we are staring our deepest fears in the face."[2] Harvard professor David Scadden concurs, "Few things make a person more engaged, authentic, and real than a serious diagnosis. People in prolonged peril . . . are without pretense."[3]

God has extended our lives for some reason (or reasons). As recipients of grace, we have the opportunity to prayerfully discern why we are still here. In this sense, living in bonus time is both a gift and a responsibility.

At the end of this chapter, I will share my new sense of purpose. Suffice to say, I have experienced both continuity (in my abilities and expertise) and discontinuity (in my professional role and physical limitations). Though the journey of discovery has not always been smooth—particularly as I've relinquished more control—my post-transplant life has been surprisingly gratifying.

WHY IS CLARITY OF PURPOSE
SO IMPORTANT?

Aristotle distinguished between two types of personal well-being: *hedonia* and *eudaimonia*. While the former Greek word relates to happiness that is short-term and shallow, the latter connects to a long-term sense of purpose.

Two examples clarify the difference. First, though few medical technicians would claim that drawing blood or collecting urine samples makes them happy (hedonia), many find significant meaning in their jobs (eudaimonia). Because they represent the entry point into the health-care system for most patients, many experience deep satisfaction in allaying patients' fears by being empathetic in an uncomfortable context. Second, while the day-to-day challenges of raising children are not always fun (hedonia), parenting is suffused with deep significance (eudaimonia).[4]

This is not to say that short-term happiness is without value. To the contrary, after a year of medical restriction, I relished eating teriyaki chicken takeout again. Writing this book has been propelled by massive doses of chocolate. Such immediate gratification presents no moral dilemma. Rather, the real problem with hedonia is its incompleteness. While buying a sports car or going on a cruise to celebrate being healthy again is perfectly understandable, neither act is sufficient to feed our souls over the long run. Pursuit of immediate pleasure quickly reaches a saturation point. While it may produce legitimate short-term happiness, it cannot address life's metaquestions.

In the film *The Bucket List*, Jack Nicholson and Morgan Freeman are terminal cancer patients thrust together as hospital roommates. Jack, married four times, is a poster child for hedonia. Morgan, a philosophical mechanic with a stable family life, represents eudaimonia. When their symptoms simultaneously go into remission, they draft a list of things they want to do before they die ("kick the bucket"). Since Jack is filthy rich, they go on an African safari, ride motorcycles on China's Great Wall, and visit the Taj Mahal.

While at the Egyptian pyramids, however, Morgan realizes that he wants to be with his wife, sons, and grandchildren before he dies. Short-term pleasurable experiences, though wonderful, don't meet his innermost need for familial love. Upset that his grand tour has been prematurely terminated, Jack gets angry. In doing so, he reveals the existence of an estranged daughter.

The film ends with Morgan being tender to his wife, enjoying a glorious feast with his sons and grandchildren, and then dying suddenly. After Jack is embraced at the funeral by Morgan's family, he seeks out his daughter and (heretofore unknown) granddaughter. We watch as Jack unconsciously migrates from hedonia to eudaimonia.

Having a purpose beyond gratifying ourselves is critical to our physical, emotional, and spiritual health. Studies show that pursuing eudaimonic well-being leads to fewer heart attacks, increased longevity, better sleep, and decreased incidence of Alzheimer's.[5] In his book *Being Mortal*, Dr. Atul Gawande encourages readers to "seek a cause beyond ourselves . . . something worth making sacrifices for. We have a need to identify purposes outside ourselves that make living feel meaningful and worthwhile."[6]

William Breitbart, chair of the department of psychiatry at Sloan Kettering Cancer Center, finds that patients who seek to end their lives via assisted suicide are not (as a group) in greater physical pain than others. Rather, they report a lack of purpose and hope. Unlike clinical depression, Dr. Breitbart writes, "meaninglessness is more of an existential concern . . . a belief that one's life has little value or purpose and is, therefore, not worth living."[7]

PROFILE: CAROLYN CROSS

Carolyn is president of Ondine Biomedical, a start-up company that manufactures a device to destroy "superbug" germs simply and cheaply. It has immense potential to save lives, particularly in developing nations with poor medical infrastructure.

Boarding a small plane in Vancouver, Canada, she was excited about her upcoming meeting with six other entrepreneurs. Shortly after takeoff, however, the aircraft began to violently shake and roll. When the pilot said that an emergency landing would be necessary, Carolyn sensed imminent disaster. She quickly texted her three kids to say goodbye: "I am proud of who you are. Love you forever. Mummy."

Carolyn felt the plane smash into the ground. Behind her, the tail sheared off; around her, flames surged. Unbuckling her seat belt, she tried to stand up but could not. Instead, she stumbled forward, breaking several teeth and injuring her skull. Nevertheless, she managed to drag herself out of the plane and onto what she discovered was a highway, just before the cabin exploded into a ball of fire.

A man driving by stopped and carried her to safety. At the hospital, Carolyn learned that she had broken several ribs and compressed her vertebrae. She and her fellow passengers were fortunate to be alive; both pilots did not survive the crash.

Living in bonus time, Carolyn is now even more committed to bring Ondine's inexpensive bacteria-killing technology to health facilities around the world: "I now have to work harder and smarter. . . . I have a very profound sense of my calling. My family understands that. I am more driven now than ever. I am determined to make a difference, even if I have to board more airplanes."[a]

[a]Sunny Dhillon, "Woman Saved from Fiery Plane Crash Consoles Grieving Hero," *Globe and Mail*, November 4, 2011, www.theglobeandmail.com/news/british-columbia /woman-saved-from-fiery-plane-crash-consoles-grieving-hero/article4248039.

HOW DO WE FIND PURPOSE?

Cancer survivors are often asked "what next?" For some, the question of purpose is relatively easy. Carolyn Cross's pre-crash desire to bring a life-saving diagnostic tool to poor nations has been enhanced with renewed intensity. Trauma reinforced her commitment and served as a catalyst to become even more focused. Her life's direction is shaped by family and her company's mission.

Likewise, Dr. Paul Kalanithi concentrated his final year on loving his wife and their newborn daughter, writing a book, and rekindling his dormant Christian faith. His widow, Lucy, later recalled:

> During the last year of his life, Paul wrote relentlessly, fueled by purpose, motivated by a ticking clock. . . . When his fingertips developed painful fissures because of his chemo, we found seamless silver-lined gloves. . . . He was determined to keep writing. . . . This book carries the urgency of racing against time, of having important things to say.[8]

Such ongoing clarity of purpose reminds me of a confident five-year-old girl Robert Fulghum describes in his book *All I Really Need to Know I Learned in Kindergarten*. Shortly after asking a group of kindergartners to organize themselves into clusters of giants, wizards, and ogres, Fulghum felt a tug on his pant leg. The girl asked, "Where do the mermaids go?" When he explained that there was no mermaid category, she asserted, "You may believe that only giants, wizards, and ogres exist, but you are wrong! I am a mermaid! Deal with it."[9]

I love this child. Having no doubt about her identity and purpose, she was a mermaid who did mermaid stuff. But for many of us entering bonus time figuring out who we are to become—and what we are to do next—is anything but clear. Gazing into the future, we see fog, not blue skies.

Timing. On a somber note, many survivors live with financial worries, chronic pain, physical limitations, unemployment, and fear of recurrence. Any of these unsettling factors can create grave uncertainty about the future. One survivor describes feeling trapped in a limbo-like existence, "The task of rebuilding your life after something as devastating as cancer can be deeply disorienting and destabilizing. I feel like I'm in no-man's land, inhabited by people like me who are neither sick nor well."[10]

Nine months post-transplant, I was far from ready to pursue clarity of purpose. Wandering through PTSD, graft-versus-host disease, and survivor's guilt, I experienced profound disequilibrium. During that time, I sought professional help, was patient with my recovery, and did not move forward prematurely. Eventually, I reached a point where I was ready to pursue eudaimonic well-being. My advice is to take all the time and get all the assistance you may need.

Three critical steps. Purpose comes into focus via three progressive phases—*surrender, assessment,* and *attentiveness.*

Surrender. For Christians the quest for direction begins with a bow of the knee. Surrender—freely choosing to place ourselves under God's will—is self-emptying and often difficult. Clearly countercultural to notions of self-assertion and independence, it requires humbling ourselves. Brother Lawrence labeled this "hearty renunciation."[11] Thankfully, our submission is not into the hands of a tyrannical abuser but to a loving Father.

This step proved surprisingly challenging for me. It took many months to slowly yield control and move to a posture of profound reliance. As I held tightly to my old identity, laying aside self-perceived "entitlements" proved difficult.

A word rarely used today—*lordship*—involves acknowledging Christ as *kyrios* (Greek for "master"). Our role? To serve as *douloi* (Greek for "slaves"). By moving into subordinated solidarity, we offer our talents, ambitions, and priorities. Life is no longer about us. The apostle Paul labeled himself a *doulos* nearly thirty times in his letters. And he encouraged us to do likewise: "You are not your own; you were bought at a price."[12]

Following his lead, for nearly a decade my morning prayers commenced, "I am your slave. I serve only one master."[13] This was my attempt to completely submit, relinquish all, and not be overly concerned about pleasing others. I must confess that it felt quite unnatural at first. Over time, it became surprisingly liberating.

Paul dove even deeper into the mystery of surrender when he utilized a second image—that of dying to self. He reflected, "I no longer live, but Christ lives in me."[14] Baptism beautifully reflects this notion. We die (descend into water), get cleansed (submerge), and resurrect to new life (lifted up). In this sense, all believers—not just those who survive near-death experiences—are living in bonus time. George Müller, an exemplary nineteenth-century disciple, captured this sentiment well: "There was a day when I died, utterly died. Died to George Müller, his opinions, preferences, tastes, and will. Died to the world, its approval or censure. Died to the approval or blame even of my brethren and friends. Since then, I have studied only to show myself approved unto God."[15]

PROFILE: TOM AND LIBBY LITTLE

While college students, Tom and Libby Little attended the Urbana 1967 Student Missions Conference. On the fifth and final day, a call was given to serve on global missions. Libby's hand shot up quickly. She had felt God's call early in the event and was ready to serve overseas. Tom was more reticent.

As Libby recalls, Tom's arm was one of the last to be raised. But he also became one of the most deeply committed. Tom yielded himself completely to God that day—his career, his future, his life.

Years passed as Tom studied optometry, but he did not forget his pledge to become a medical missionary. He married Libby, and they made Afghanistan their home for thirty-five years. Together, they raised three daughters and endured three bloody wars.

In 2010, Tom and nine medical compatriots were traveling in a remote northern valley to provide care. For years, the Taliban had allowed such teams unimpeded access. But not that day. The ten were lined up and shot execution style. Because of his decades of service and self-sacrifice, Tom was one of fifteen recipients of the 2011 Presidential Medal of Freedom, America's highest civilian award.

When Libby spoke to a new generation of students at Urbana the next year, she said, "Tom didn't die in Afghanistan in 2010. He died at Urbana 1967." By raising his hand forty-five years earlier, he had surrendered his life fully to God. His commitment had held steady.[a]

[a]Rod Nordland, "Gunmen Kill Medical Aid Workers in Afghanistan," *New York Times*, August 7, 2010, www.nytimes.com/2010/08/08/world/asia/08afghan.html.

Assessment. Our search for clarity of purpose continues with assessment. This entails taking stock of existing responsibilities, evaluating our physical capabilities, reflecting on our sense of calling, and listening to trusted advisers.

First, we identify our precancer responsibilities such as caring for a loved one or completing a project. In such situations, purpose finds us rather than vice versa. While cancer may interrupt the flow of our lives, core duties abide. Of course, physical, mental, or emotional limitations may reduce our capacity to serve.

I marvel at Andrea Thomas, who moved with her family from Michigan to rebuild InterVarsity's campus ministry in Texas, Oklahoma, and Arkansas. She served with her husband as co-regional directors, a first for the ministry. Life was more than full as they hired new staff, raised funds, and planted new chapters at universities across the region. Andrea was so talented that she was one of only fourteen staff (out of 1,700) selected to participate in a two-year prospective senior leaders' cohort.

Andrea was diagnosed with breast cancer at age thirty-five and was given a 50 percent chance of survival. She worried about her husband and their three children—ages eight, six, and two. For nearly a year, she underwent multiple surgeries and intense chemo. As she returned to work part-time, she began five years of hormone therapy. That difficult period was marked with chemo brain, deep fatigue, and emotional fluctuations.

As she slowly emerged from the cancer pit, she found it relatively easy to regain a clear sense of calling. Her dance card was filled with existing commitments to family and ministry. Minimal time was spent pondering new goals and priorities—she already knew what she had to do. Today, thirteen years later with two kids in college, she is identifying a new vocational purpose.

Second, we reassess our physical capabilities. With our altered bodies, we may struggle with self-confidence, strength, and stamina. Our ability to concentrate may be impaired. I have had to come to grips with a variety of deficits and ailments. While such reflection is not enjoyable, it is crucial. As we adjust to our new limitations, we may experience varying levels of sadness. There is real loss here.

As I've sought clarity of purpose, some things can be ruled out. For example, I ought not serve in a sunny climate (hence Seattle is perfect). I should not run a large organization (my lack of verbal filters could cause problems and my memory is not as sharp). Joint soreness limits my ability to lift and carry.

Third, we assess our sense of calling. What passions, skills, and experiences give us energy and joy? In an oft-quoted phrase, Frederick Buechner advises, "The place God calls you to is the place where your deep gladness and the world's deep hunger meet."[16] Post-treatment, what is your "deep gladness?" It may be a continuation or something entirely new. Take time to reflect. There are so many options. Some teach refugees, launch a new venture, or volunteer at a food bank. Others create art, love toddlers, or write.

Living an unexamined life means falling lazily back into old habits rather than acting out of conviction. Cancer provides a rare opportunity—a gift really—to redefine our personal narrative. We can start anew by being intentional about things that really matter.[17] That which previously engaged our imagination may no longer do so. We may now realize that our former dream was ill-defined. Bonus time gives us the chance to declutter, filter, and refine.

Valerie Yates was forty-nine when cancer struck. While successful as a marketing director, she used her recovery period to reflect: "I suppose, when you stop seeing yourself as immortal, you ask, 'What am I going to do for the rest of my life that will have meaning?'" Realizing how toxic her work environment had become, she assessed what gave her joy. Her conclusion: "Being at home with people gathered around my table, enjoying themselves." So, she quit her job and opened her house as a bed and breakfast. She is entirely pleased with the change.[18]

For some, calling is rooted in either paying it back (to those who helped us) or paying it forward (to others in need). J. C., a young New York financier, was on a trajectory to be at the top of her profession when she was sidelined by a devastating cancer. While in recovery, she reevaluated her priorities and decided to become a doctor. While her decision did not appear to be terribly practical—it meant quitting a secure job, taking undergraduate science courses, and then attending medical school—she faithfully acted on her convictions. Today, J. C. is an emergency room doctor, paying it both back and ahead.[19]

Fourth, we avidly seek the wise counsel of spouses, pastors, licensed counselors, and close friends. Which of our attributes do they observe hardwired in us? Where do they see our temperaments, experiences, and interests intersecting? In what ways have we changed post-treatment? We ask for their opinions because what is obvious to them may be a blind spot for us. At times, I'm completely amazed by how others see me. My capacity for self-delusion is remarkable.

Attentiveness. In his book *The Attentive Life*, Leighton Ford defines attentiveness as "not so much doing for God as paying attention to what God is doing."[20] This means slowing down, listening, watching, and reflecting.

For extroverted, fast-paced addicts like me, this is truly difficult. None of the spiritual disciplines commonly associated with attentiveness—solitude, retreats, sabbath rest, and journal writing—come naturally for me. But over the years patterns have become integral parts of my life. Monks describe these habits as a "rule of life." While their routines certainly contain greater intentionality than mine, I am inspired by their example. Creating space for contemplative listening is invaluable.

When cancer struck, I felt compelled to exercise greater attentiveness. If I wanted to discern God's purpose in bonus time, I had to carve out significant nondistractible time. So, I have subsequently added a second walk each day and extended my morning quiet times.

I also embrace a nascent movement known as a "technology sabbath" launched by a group of Jewish professionals. Highlighted in the *Harvard Business Review*, they recommend a weekly twenty-four-hour break from email, computers, and the internet (some add cell phones and TV). Tiffany Shlain writes, "The technology we've created takes something away from us: being present, focused, and in the moment."[21]

A friend of mine is the chief financial officer of a large multinational company. Despite an incredibly demanding schedule, he is somehow able to feed his soul through reflective writing and retreats of solitude. Truly one of the most spiritually attentive people I know, he schedules time for contemplation. When we talk, it feels as though I'm interacting with a spiritual director rather than a corporate executive. His insights are amazing. Because he listens so carefully to God, he also hears others well.

Cancer forced me to step down from a fast-paced leadership position and move into a quiet space. While many survivors simply don't have this luxury—work, family, and financial obligations continue to vie for time—God graciously understands that context matters. He only asks us to do our best with what we have.

My new purpose. The journey to my bonus-time calling was not smooth. Moving into a posture of surrender proved challenging. Reassessing my "deepest gladness," values, and skills—and seeking the advice of select friends—was a tad easier. Journaling and long walks were the greatest clarifiers in my quest.

Over time, it became clear that I should invest in next-generation leaders. Consequently, my core activities are now mentoring and teaching—actions that blend the needs of others, my deepest gladness, and my sense of direction. This clarity did not arrive overnight but only through a prolonged process of surrender, assessment, and attentiveness to the Holy Spirit.

Mary has been on a parallel journey in defining her new sense of direction. Motivated by a desire to learn firsthand about the challenges of poverty and addiction, she currently volunteers at a nonprofit that provides transitional housing for homeless families. In addition, she serves breakfast to methadone patients through our church.

I pray that you will discover God's purposes for the next season of your life. Living in bonus time with clarity is exciting. May your sharpened sense of calling allow you to say yes to the right things and let other opportunities slide by. It is a remarkable way to live.

REFLECTION QUESTIONS

1. Is defining a clear sense of purpose difficult for you? If so, how?

2. Do you struggle with surrendering your aspirations to God? If so, why?

3. What comes to mind as you think about the processes of assessment and attentiveness? What steps have you taken?

What actions do you feel God leading you toward in the future?

4. Reflect on Psalm 18:1-6, 16-19.

> I love you, LORD, my strength.
> The LORD is my rock, my fortress and my deliverer;
>> my God is my rock, in whom I take refuge,
>> my shield and the horn of my salvation, my
>>> stronghold.
> I called to the LORD, who is worthy of praise,
>> and I have been saved from my enemies.
> The cords of death entangled me;
>> the torrents of destruction overwhelmed me.
> The cords of the grave coiled around me;
>> the snares of death confronted me.
> In my distress I called to the LORD;
>> I cried to my God for help.
> From his temple he heard my voice;
>> my cry came before him, into his ears. . . .
> He reached down from on high and took hold of me;
>> he drew me out of deep waters.
> He rescued me from my powerful enemy,
>> from my foes, who were too strong for me.
> They confronted me in the day of my disaster,
>> but the LORD was my support.
> He brought me out into a spacious place;
>> he rescued me because he delighted in me.

10

REDEEMING TIME

Somebody should tell us, right at the start of our lives,
that we are dying. Then we might live life to the limit, every
minute of every day. There are only so many tomorrows.

POPE PAUL VI

No matter what happens—whether the cancer never
flares up again or whether you die—the important thing
is that the days that you've had you will have lived.

GILDA RADNER

Today is only one day in all the days that will ever be.
But what will happen in all the other days that ever
come can depend on what you do today.

ERNEST HEMINGWAY

I don't want to get to the end of my life and find that I have just
lived the length of it. I want to have lived the width of it as well.

DIANE ACKERMAN

B E DILIGENT HOW YOU WALK [LIVE]. Wise people redeem the time." So advises the apostle Paul.[1]

In this chapter, we will explore what it means to "redeem time." As cancer survivors living in bonus time, we have been given a second chance not only to redefine our purpose in life but to steward our remaining days wisely.

Most people tend to view the future as having a long trajectory. But a cancer diagnosis causes time horizons to shrink. Researchers label this recalibration an *existential slap*.[2] Abruptly shifting from expansive time to abbreviated time can be jolting. For someone like me, who used to plan vacations two years in advance, the adjustment has been profound. Such loss of control is often difficult to absorb.

Psychologists have coined a phrase—*life span theory*—to contrast the radically different perspectives of those who expect to live a long time versus those who do not. The latter group includes the elderly, the ill, and those in life-threatening situations (such as Chinese during the bird flu outbreak or West Africans when Ebola spread).[3]

Young adults—who possess a seemingly endless time horizon— prize having novel experiences, meeting new people, and learning new things. Priorities include achievement and exploration.[4] By contrast, those who have come face-to-face with death live more in the now, covet existing relationships, and seek to repeat emotionally satisfying experiences. Unlike twentysomethings, most would rather dine with a close friend than a published author.[5]

Exactly how we redeem time has much to do with our stage of life. Moses crafted Psalm 90—the only poem (of 150) attributed to him—probably as an old man. Of all the themes this great leader could have chosen, he reflected on lifespan. His best remembered words come in the form of a prayer: "Teach us to number our days, that we may gain a heart of wisdom."[6]

Cancer survivors grasp the import of Moses' petition "to number our days." We yearn to use our remaining time well and not be sidetracked by trivialities. Fully aware of our finiteness, we seek to focus on what's truly important. Our quest is a "heart of wisdom." As Benjamin Franklin remarked: "Do you love life? Then don't squander time, for time is the stuff life is made of."[7]

For many survivors, the prospect of mortality profoundly affects the lifespan calculus. Some cancers are only temporarily beaten back. Others technically go away, but recurrence is an ever-present danger. Still others are completely healed, but collateral damage done by poisonous drugs, radiation, and surgery may trigger new life-threatening maladies. Regular appointments with my oncologist and dermatologist provide reminders of my limited remaining years. I appreciate Billy Graham's response when asked what surprised him most about life: "Its brevity."[8]

How we "redeem time" and "number our days" is, in part, influenced by how we assess our expected lifespan. Shortly before discovering that his cancer was terminal, Dr. Paul Kalanithi decided to allocate his remaining time as follows: "Tell me three months, I'd spend time with my family. Tell me one year, I'd write a book. Give me ten years, I'd get back to treating diseases."[9]

OPPORTUNITIES FOR GROWTH

The ancient Greek language employed two words to define time. The first, *chronos*, describes clock or calendar time—measured linearly in seconds, minutes, hours, days, and years. The second, *kairos*, points to life's grand moments when we say, "my whole life changed when . . ." While the former is scientifically objective and relates to quantity of time, the latter is subjectively rich with meaning and refers to quality of time.[10]

As cancer survivors living in bonus time, we have a rich opportunity to increase our sense of kairos. Rather than living mechanically day to day, the gate is open for us to gain a heart of wisdom and joy. An old French saying nicely captures the idea: "God works in moments" (*en peu d'heure Dieu labeure*).[11] A terminally ill British patient recently echoed this sentiment: "I realised I preferred a short life lived well than a long life lived badly."[12] In other words, if forced to choose, she opted for kairos over chronos.

This is not to say that chronos is bad. To the contrary, it is essential. When Mary and I celebrate the date of my transplant with a birthday cake and candles, we are acknowledging its importance. (I must add that it was simply smashing to be three years old again.) Chronos is like an empty glass. While it does not satisfy our thirst directly, it provides the vehicle for water to be served. Kairos is the water.

After being hit by the existential slap of cancer, many of us regret the amount of chronos we wasted prior to diagnosis. But we can't go back. We are different people now. The good news is that we have been given future chronos. This presents us with the opportunity to redeem time in at least four ways. First, we learn to savor each moment. Second, we focus more on relationships and less on achievements. Third, we clean up our messes and find greater freedom. Finally, having received so much help from others, we slingshot this goodwill ahead to benefit others.

Savor moments. My precancer life was pell-mell. So much in a hurry to charge the next hill, I sadly missed thousands (millions?) of special moments. And now? When I'm taken aback by the autumn glow of a tree, I pause to capture the moment in a photo so I can enjoy it anew later. When a puppy walks by, I bend down to ruffle its fur. When a nephew or niece calls, I don't watch the clock. When Mary asks to spend an extra night camping, I try to accommodate. When two driving routes are options, I often take the slower and more scenic one.

Cherishing the here and now is a grace from God. Being too focused on the future blinds us to what is priceless in this moment. Cancer teaches us that strolling is sometimes better than sprinting. Flexibility becomes a virtue.

Many of us remember Shannon Miller, gold medal gymnast at the 1996 Olympics. Fifteen years later, at the age of thirty-four, she was diagnosed with ovarian cancer. Her time perspective completely changed: "I used to fly through life. I didn't take time to savor it. I was always go, go, go. Now I understand the importance of really taking time to appreciate every moment."[13]

PROFILE: AN ANONYMOUS MONK

In a striking reflection, a Nebraskan monk looked back on his long life. After spending years of not relishing each day—rather deferring gratification until tomorrow—he wished that he had lived more in the present tense.

His words serve as a warning for those of us who are so driven that we speed past God's handiwork—some of which may only be seen at a slower pace. Self-discipline has its place, but so does celebrating each day. He wrote the following:

> If I had my life to live over again . . . I would climb more mountains, swim more rivers, and watch more sunsets. . . .
>
> I would eat more ice cream and less beans.

You see, I'm one of those people who lives . . . sensibly hour after hour, day after day. Oh, I've had my moments, and if I had to do it over again I would have more of them.

In fact, I'd try to have nothing else, just moments, one after another, instead of living so many years ahead each day. I've been one of those people who never go anywhere without a thermometer, a hot-water bottle, a raincoat, aspirin, and a parachute.

If I had to do it over again . . . I would travel lighter. . . .

I would start barefooted earlier in the spring and stay that way later in the fall. . . .

I would ride on more merry-go-rounds and pick more daisies.[a]

[a]Monk, quoted by Chuck Swindoll, *Three Steps Forward, Two Steps Back* (New York: Bantam, 1982), 42-43.

Love deeply. Most cancer survivors experience a fascinating trade-off between achievement and relationships. Studies show that success becomes less important while loving others ascends as a priority.[14] This has certainly been my experience. Moving from a fast-paced leadership role, I now mentor younger leaders. For someone with my driven personality to become deeply enmeshed in their successes and sorrows has been an unexpected pleasure. Now that I am more available to others, I feel deeply connected and enriched.

The last chapter referenced *The Bucket List*, a film starring Morgan Freeman and Jack Nicholson. Its simple moral is that while activities, adventures, and achievements are all well and good, loving deeply is more satisfying and enduring. Saying "I love you" is of greater value than adding another trophy on the wall. Kate Bowler, a Duke professor with stage 4 cancer, got it exactly right when she hung a huge sign for her husband: "YOU ARE MY BUCKET LIST."[15]

A Harvard University study, conducted over eight decades, concludes that close relationships are more determinative of good health and psychological contentment than accomplishments. Indeed, being connected to others is a better predictor of long life than one's genes, IQ, or social class. Notes the director of the study, "Tending to your relationships is a form of self-care."[16] When those we love take priority over success, fortune, and fame, we are happier and healthier.

In his song "Live Like You Were Dying," Tim McGraw tells of a man who receives a terminal diagnosis. This closely parallel's McGraw's real-life father, who contracted a brain tumor and died nine months later. The man decides to go skydiving, mountain climbing, and bull riding. But the heart of the lyrics home in on relationships: "And I loved deeper, and I spoke sweeter, and I gave forgiveness I'd been denying."[17] He then became the kind of husband and friend he had never been before.

With our remaining time on earth, most of us yearn to be with those we love. As priorities are resorted, this may mean delaying projects or placing less emphasis on our careers. It may also include taking longer family vacations, enjoying walks with loved ones, and hosting meals with old friends. My relationship with Mary has certainly entered a season of renaissance. The bonus time we experience is to be treasured. Every conversation is special.

Author John Claypool tells a moving story of his four-year-old daughter, Laura, who later died of leukemia. One night, he became frustrated at bedtime when she—like so many other kids her age—wouldn't settle down. Moments later he noticed her standing at his door. A tad angered, he asked, "What do you want me to do?" She walked over, grabbed his hand, and said, "Nothing, Daddy. I just want to be close to you."[18]

Live freely. Redeeming time means taking tangible steps to disencumber our lives. This includes getting right with God, cleaning up relational messes, unshackling ourselves from bad habits, and detaching from possessions that weigh us down. In other words, we take care of unfinished matters that hold us back and hurt others.

"Fessing up" to the Lord signifies repenting of past sins. It may also include reaching out to those we've offended. When diagnosed with bladder cancer, former Vice President Hubert Humphrey reconciled with several political rivals, including Richard Nixon and Jesse Jackson. He told the latter, "If I were to die this year, I wouldn't want to leave any unfinished business. . . . I want to get it straight. At a time like this you are forced to deal with your irreducible essence. . . . And what I have concluded . . . is that we must forgive each other, and redeem each other and then move on."[19]

Broken relationships bruise our souls. Author Malachy McCourt wisely warns, "Holding a grudge is like drinking poison and expecting the other person to die."[20] Reengaging positively with those who have provoked us to bitterness in the past can be liberating. Forgiveness is another amazing antidote.

About a decade ago, I took Jesus' command to love my enemies[21] seriously by praying every Friday for a brief list of people for whom I harbored ill feelings. One person remained on the list for eight years before the last vestige of bile left my soul. My prayer wasn't that they would improve but that the Lord would bless them. This spiritual discipline changed my heart over time.

Living free also means being unfettered from others' expectations. Life is simply too short to constantly bend to other's opinions. As a people pleaser, this tendency has been an ongoing challenge for me. Post-treatment, it has been incredibly liberating to care less. How I wish I had discovered this freedom earlier in life. Mary has been pleasantly surprised by my newfound forthrightness, a gift of bonus time.

Shortly before his death, Steve Jobs delivered a brilliant commencement address at Stanford University. Advising graduates not to worry about external expectations, he said, "These things just fall away in the face of death, leaving only what is truly important. Remembering that you are going to die is the best way I know to avoid the trap of thinking you have something to lose. You are already naked. . . . Your time is limited, so don't waste it living someone else's life."[22]

Those who live freely don't get sidetracked by small stuff. I find myself being less bothered by slow drivers, cranky neighbors, waiting in line, or an underperforming sports team. By focusing on kairos, temporary annoyances tend to roll off my shoulders.

I also engage less with social media. Seeing the future as time limited, I am not as drawn to reading the latest post. Research shows that reducing our computer usage and TV viewing significantly decreases the odds of depression.[23] When it comes to politics, I now try to cap my reading and viewing at one hour per day. Given the colorful personalities involved, I can easily get sucked into matters that may seem critical today but fade from the news cycle a week later. While it is important to be aware, it is unwise to be consumed.

Do good. As cancer survivors, we have the privilege to share what God's presence means in our lives. Shortly after my year of isolation ended, I volunteered to colead an Alpha class at my church. Alpha provides a series of short videos for spiritual seekers who consider themselves outside the Christian faith. Why did I make this a priority? Sensing my mortality and glimpsing the afterlife, I felt more compelled to share the good news with others.

Likewise, we are graced with the opportunity to serve others in need (e.g., immigrants, children, elderly, and disabled). Doing good also includes being available to patients entering the cancer tunnel. What an incredible honor to be supportive when they experience their first existential slap. The bond can be profound.

Henri Nouwen rhetorically asks, "How many people run to where others are suffering?"[24] The obvious answer is not many. But as survivors, we have good reasons to be at the front of the line. Kate Bowler intuits that her cancer mysteriously connects her to others in distress: "I notice the look of exhaustion on the young mom's face at the grocery store and help her with her cart. I stop to talk to the homeless man sitting on the corner. I give money away more freely, less begrudgingly."[25]

Perhaps the greatest service we can offer is simply listening well. Caring for my mentees, I hope that they find a warm heart and sensitive ears. Their words matter. When one is under water emotionally, it is my privilege to attend, counsel, and encourage. Empathy grows out of the soil of personal pain. As survivors, we have a reservoir of grit to give to others. Serving is not only the right thing to do, it is good for our souls. We can either draw from this well or let the water stagnate. Tim Keller counsels, "Suffering is almost a prerequisite if we are going to be of much use to other people, especially when they go through their own trials. Adversity makes us far more compassionate. We become more tender-hearted."[26]

PROFILE: KATE GRANGER

At twenty-nine, Kate was a British geriatric doctor at the top of her craft. However, it all came crashing down when a kidney failed while on vacation in California.

After several rounds of tests, a junior doctor entered her hospital room and blurted out one sentence: "The MRI scan shows that you have cancer and it has spread." Kate recalls, "He couldn't leave the room fast enough. I felt scarred by that experience." She vowed to treat her patients better.

Kate had an incurable tumor. The average length of survival was fourteen months. As a doctor of the elderly, she was familiar with end-of-life issues but never expected to apply these lessons to herself at such an early age.

Friends expressed surprise when Kate returned to work. After all, it was a stressful job at a public hospital. Her rationale? "Working has given me a focus again, and I think I still have a great deal to give—probably more than before my own illness."

She felt a strong call to serve others in need: it gave her purpose and great satisfaction. Elderly patients loved her. Working three days a week, she continued to push herself until sidelined by fatigue.

Kate surprised her doctors by living another five years. In that time, she and her husband raised nearly $320,000 for their local cancer center. In her honor, England's National Health Service created the Kate Granger Award for Compassionate Care. She was also made a fellow of the Royal College of Physicians in recognition of her love for elderly patients.[a]

[a]Kate Granger, "Terminal Cancer: How to Live with Dying," *Guardian*, September 19, 2012, www.theguardian.com/lifeandstyle/2012/sep/19/terminal-cancer-how-to-live-with-dying.

Paul urges us to "redeem time" and Moses prays for a "heart of wisdom." After surviving cancer's existential slap, we are privileged to faithfully steward our remaining days by celebrating moments, loving without reservation, living freely, and serving others. This is the formula for a rich life, no matter how long it lasts.

REFLECTION QUESTIONS

1. How has cancer affected your sense of time and relationships?

2. What (or better who) is on your bucket list?

3. What holds you back from living more freely?

4. Reflect on excerpts from Psalm 90. How do its insights apply to you?

> A thousand years in your sight
>   are like a day that has just gone by,
>   or like a watch in the night.
> Yet you sweep people away in the sleep of death—
>   they are like the new grass of the morning:
> In the morning it springs up new,
>   but by evening it is dry and withered. . . .
> Our days may come to seventy years,
>   or eighty, if our strength endures;
> yet the best of them are but trouble and sorrow,
>   for they quickly pass, and we fly away. . . .
> Teach us to number our days
>   that we may gain a heart of wisdom. . . .
> Satisfy us in the morning with your unfailing love,
>   that we may sing for joy and be glad all our days.
> Make us glad for as many days as you have afflicted us,
>   for as many years as we have seen trouble.

11

WONDER

How do I not become a hollow soul? Never lose the wonder.

MARGARET FEINBERG

Wonder is the thing that makes it possible to sing about amazing grace instead of simply saying that God is gracious.

JESSE HILL

Scars may heal, blood counts may normalize, years may pass. But never again will the simple act of waking up to a normal, boring day as a healthy individual be taken for granted.

ALLISON, CANCER SURVIVOR

When it's over, I want to say: All my life I was a bride married to amazement.

MARY OLIVER

A s I welcomed Easter parishioners, I noted the normalcy of the morning. A typical Seattle April day with high clouds and a slight chill, families arrived in three generational clusters. Teens looked as if they should have stayed in bed. The day, however, was anything but ordinary for me. After a year of physical isolation, I was serving as a greeter.

For far too long I had not been allowed to touch anyone due to risk of infection. Yet, here I was, grabbing hands as eagerly as Teddy Roosevelt at his inaugural. The realization that I had no need for hand sanitizer brought a quiet smile. A simple tactile act—extending an open hand to others—took on a sacramental character. Like the lepers touched by Jesus, my long ostracism was over. Not only had I been physically healed but I was now able to socially reconnect.

Wonder captures our attention and pierces our souls. Typically, it involves something grand. But for cancer survivors its scope is widened to include the everyday "normal" that has been denied for a long time—like holding a baby or walking in the rain. This is one of cancer's "gifts." While healthy people generally experience wonder only in the extraordinary, those of us who have been deathly sick also sense it in the ordinary. No doubt my sense of wonder that first Easter was special.

Though a rather elusive concept to define, three attributes of wonder stand out. First, it involves experiencing something larger than ourselves. Second, it engenders epiphanies. And third, it represents a sensation that we desperately want to sustain.[1]

SOMETHING GREATER THAN OURSELVES

Synonyms for wonder include *transcendence*, *astonishment*, and *sublimity*.[2] Wonder makes us gasp, causing us to say, "Oh my." Looking over the rim of Oregon's Crater Lake for the first time was one of those moments for me. It simply took my breath away. Formed after a mountain imploded, the resultant caldera is the deepest lake in the United States and one of the most pristine in the world. Not only massive, its waters are an other-worldly sapphire blue.

Wonder may be experienced while walking a shoreline, looking into the galaxy, watching a newborn enter the world, listening to incredible music, huddling during a lightning storm, or musing in front of a masterpiece. Astronauts report an astonishing sensation as they look back to earth.[3] The most incredible places of the ancient world are referred to simply as the *seven wonders*.

Near-death experiences often elicit wonder. After being hit by something larger than ourselves—be it cancer, an accident, or an addiction—we ask ourselves how we survived something so powerful. Recognizing that much was outside our control, we are thrilled simply to be living.

As a child, I loved a game called Labyrinth. It was a wooden maze with two knobs, and I tried to steer a steel marble past thirty-six holes and out the back of the box. Coordinating the pitch and tilt of the board was very challenging. A slight miscalculation would end the game. In the month following my transplant, I imagined myself in a revised version where I was the marble and each hole represented death. Having no access to the knobs, I watched as my metaphorical marble slowly snaked past hole after hole and finally exited the box to survival. Though incredibly frightening at the time, I now look back in stunned wonder.

Survivors experience an astonishing range of emotions. Prior chapters discussed negative feelings such as guilt, fear, anger, and confusion. But there are positive sentiments as well—such as joy, gratitude, and clarity. At the oddest times I find myself blurting out loud: "I'm alive!"

PROFILE: SOPHIA ANAGNOSTOU

Sophia was twelve years old when diagnosed with leukemia. Her mother, Tara, recalls being "numb with fear." Over the course of three years, treatments included chemotherapy, spinal taps, red cell and platelet transfusions, and multiple surgeries.

Mostly restricted to home, Sophia sadly remembers, "If I went somewhere, I'd get stared at" due to hair loss, skin pallor, and surgical face mask. "Every day I was saying 'why me?' I was depressed. I missed my friends." She could not attend school her entire seventh-grade year.

Now well on her way to recovery, Sophia celebrates the wonder of life: "I'm grateful to be able to run and go outside and eat in restaurants. All the things I never used to think about, I think about now." She has even composed a song titled "Strength Is in the Soul." In it, she credits her family, caregivers, friends, and God.

Tara also has been bolstered by her Christian faith. Reflecting on wonder, she observes, "My whole outlook on life is different now. There is a lot of beauty in our lives to appreciate the little things and the things that are authentic and real. It opens your eyes to a lot of truths that were probably in front of me the whole time, and I just didn't realize it." She says she's been helped by her faith in God, her parents, her community, and Sophia's doctor.[a]

Sophia's video is a must see. What an incredible celebration of life![b]

[a]Stacy Simon, "Childhood Leukemia Survivor Finds Beauty in Life," *American Cancer Society*, September 26, 2016, www.cancer.org/latest-news/childhood-leukemia -survivor-finds-beauty-in-life.html.

[b]Sophia Anagnostou with Anita Kruse, "Strength Is in the Soul," YouTube, May 22, 2016, www.youtube.com/watch?v=Ya_N2MuwaDo.

EPIPHANIES

An epiphany is a kairos moment when something transcendent is revealed to us. We may experience it as an illuminating insight. Such events, both uplifting and humbling, are the epitome of spiritual wonder. That which is awe-inspiring becomes embedded in our souls.

My cancer journey has inspired several such epiphanies. I learned that God is with me in dark days of pain, that even when not understanding his ways I trust him, that I no longer fear death, that I am far grittier than before, that bonus time is filled with purpose, and that Mary loves me much more than I ever imagined.

An appropriate response to transcendence is stillness, even submission. Ralph Waldo Emerson observed, "All egotism vanishes. I am nothing."[4] Abraham Maslow described it as "being graced."[5] This has certainly been my response. The sense of Jesus as my friend (which he is) has become secondary to the realization that he is more formidable than I had previously imagined. My faith has been tempered by a holy sense of awe.

The foremost epiphany in Scripture is the revelation of Jesus when he came to earth. Many churches host a Feast of the Epiphany after Christmas to celebrate his entrance into a dark world. Paul's journey to Damascus is another account. On his way to persecute Christians, a bright light knocked him to the ground where—blinded—he heard Jesus' voice. This humbling event shattered him to the core, transforming him from harshest foe to staunchest advocate. A third example is Jesus' transfiguration in front of Peter, John, and James. Seeing him through new eyes, they heard God's voice from heaven and absorbed his elevated standing vis-à-vis Moses and Elijah. Like Paul, they were deeply humbled by the event.[6]

What ties these stories together is the concept of *liminal space*—an expanded sense of place where we experience God with one foot in the material world and the other in a spiritual world. Earlier, I shared how I sensed the Lord's presence in unique and powerful ways following my transplant. I never want to lose what Jean Pierre de Caussade, a French mystic, labels "the sacrament of the present moment." C. S. Lewis created an entire imaginary liminal world, entered through a wardrobe, named Narnia.[7]

Kate Bowler was a thirty-five-year-old rising academic star when diagnosed with colon cancer. She describes her liminal moment: "When I was sure I was going to die, I didn't feel angry. I felt loved. I uncovered something like a secret about faith. At the time I should have felt abandoned by God, I was not reduced to ashes. I felt like I was floating."[8]

Bowler's experience is not unique. Thousands of people with near-death experiences testify to feeling a stunning sense of peace, safety, joy, and love.[9] Richard Tedeschi recalls one of his patients whose helicopter was shot down during the Vietnam War. As the craft plummeted amid chaotic gunfire, "A great peace came over him. He felt connected to everyone, even enemy soldiers. He has tried to remain true to that connection he felt long ago. That became a guideline for his life."[10]

CULTIVATING WONDER

The idea that wonder can be cultivated seems oxymoronic. Is it possible to tame the untamable? To capture the elusive? To organize the wild? The short answer is no. We don't catch wonder. It catches us. That said, I believe that it is possible to put ourselves in wonder's way.

We cultivate wonder by pursuing God. Since my transplant, I have tried to live with childlike wonder in God's presence. Refusing to accept the notion—as some teach—that such feelings are like a passing adrenaline rush, I expectantly put myself in God's way via morning quiet times, solo walks, journaling, and worshiping with others.

In her book *Wonderstruck: Awaken to the Nearness of God*, cancer survivor Margaret Feinberg encourages us to look beyond the messy details of our daily lives and to perceive what God is doing all around us. She recommends that we literally pray for wonder each morning, asking him to enlarge our eyes to see more. Like children, she encourages us to enter each day with a sense of anticipation, interacting with God in freshness rather than thoughtless routine.[11]

Reading Scriptures afresh is another pathway to God. The psalmist affirms, "Your testimonies are wonderful."[12] Ignatius Loyola, founder of the Jesuits, taught members of his religious order to use all five senses when reading a passage. For example, when Jesus raised Lazarus from the dead, how did the tomb smell? What did Lazarus's unwrapped face look like? How did his three-day-old strips of cloth feel? What sound did the stone make when it was rolled away? Stanford professor Tanya Luhrmann finds that those who read Scripture this way are much more likely to enter liminal space than those who merely hear a lecture on the same passage.[13] Michael Card labels this practice "informed imagination."[14]

Likewise, Sunday worship should be as much about our hearts as our heads. Wonder happens when we pursue God experientially in song, meditation, and prayer. For example, when we contemplate the doctrine of the atonement in a sermon, we also need to experience it in musical worship. Responding in astonishment at God's incredible love for us and Jesus' radical sacrifice in dying for our sins, we fall to our knees in adoration. One reaction elicits mental assent while the other provokes tears of gratitude.[15]

That is what I experienced during my first post-transplant Easter service. Lyrics of virtually every song pierced my heart. Death and resurrection were highly personalized and fresh ("I was dead but am now alive"). My sense of wonder was off the charts and my informed imagination was in fifth gear. Every part of my being—body, spirit, and mind—was fully engaged.

We cultivate wonder by slowing down. Prior to my second cancer, I ran hard as InterVarsity's president for fourteen years. While I mostly loved the job, I often found myself thirsty for solitude and rest. Over time, Sundays became holy. I simply did nothing work related. Even email was verboten. Planning three-week vacations evolved over time—one week to crash, one to regain strength, and one to rejuvenate creativity. In my tenth year I was granted a three-month sabbatical, which was a remarkable gift. I returned to work reenergized. In other words, I learned how to slow down despite an over-the-top job.

Currently, I'm employed thirty hours a week. This allows extended quiet times and walks. I also have more flexibility to read, think, see friends, and volunteer. My extreme extroversion has been tempered by a newly discovered introverted side. All of this is good. Certainly, this pace is more appropriate for someone at my stage of life. Many survivors aren't so fortunate—work and family responsibilities are far greater.

Leighton Ford reminds us that "hurry is the great enemy of the life of the spirit."[16] When we quiet ourselves—whether for one hour or one day a week—our eyes are opened to the wonder all around us. Being deprived of awe is to our souls the equivalent of sun deprivation to our health. As Jesus said, we do not live by bread alone but by the wonders of God's provision.[17] In his book *Essentialism*, Greg McKeown encourages us to consciously reduce the clutter in our lives so we can more richly experience that which is truly significant.[18]

We cultivate wonder by encountering nature. A ferry ride from our home, the Olympic Peninsula is an incredibly diverse ecosystem of mountains, seashores, and rain forests. To say that Mary and I love this vast expanse of wonder would be a gross understatement. We regularly skip over to hike and camp. I often scan the stars in the middle of the night with a pair of binoculars.

One of our favorite destinations is a five-mile sand spit with a historic lighthouse at the end with Mounts Baker and Victoria (Canada) in full view. Harbor seals bob up and down in the water. The area contains a national preserve with two hundred species of migratory birds. When Scripture urges us to "stop and consider God's wonders" and to "be stunned and amazed," I have little difficulty doing so.[19]

Nature points to our Creator. It reminds us of his immensity and beauty. Talking with an atheist friend, the Olympic Peninsula is one of the best points in presenting my faith. Surely, spending time outdoors keeps our sense of wonder alive. It stirs our souls and lifts our spirits. We can also experience nature in simpler day-to-day ways such as gardening, walking the dog, watching a sunset, tending a birdfeeder, or enjoying a picnic.

Researchers have found that spending even a single minute in a grove of trees is enough to elicit awe.[20] For me, the equivalent is picking wild blackberries every August. This revisitation of a favorite childhood experience is simply wonderful (particularly since I couldn't do so for two years). Leighton Ford tells the story of Louis Agassiz, a Harvard biology professor, who told friends that he had spent his summer traveling. When asked where, he responded that "he had only got halfway across his own backyard."[21]

Margaret Feinberg regularly walks the same pathway near her home every morning. Over time her excursions sadly degenerated into a bland exercise routine. Realizing this, she began to pray for her eyes to be opened to wonder around her. Then something special occurred. She began to see so much more:

> The sight of a white butterfly landing on a lavender flower petal. A sunset's last wild burst of beauty. The sweet fragrance of the forest. Just a few weeks ago, I came upon a deer that had just given birth to two fawns. I watched awestruck as these babies took some of their first wobbly steps. How did I walk the same trail more than a thousand times and not notice such details or encounter such unforgettable moments? I don't know.[22]

We cultivate wonder by sharing our story. Research shows that sharing our cancer journeys with others can significantly improve our outlook.[23] Ways to express ourselves abound—talking, painting, crafting poems, or composing music. Even reflective journaling can lift our spirits. Writing this book has been remarkably cathartic for me. Most mornings, I can hardly wait to get to the computer.

PROFILE: CHRISSY DUNN

Chrissy was forty-six and a mother of three when she was diagnosed with stage 3 pancreatic cancer. "My family's world was shattered," she recalls. Oncologists couldn't surgically remove the tumor because it was intertwined with veins and arteries. She was given a 6 percent chance of survival.

She reflects, "The first time I walked into the chemotherapy room I was scared out of my mind, but it became a place of comfort. Now I miss the people in the infusion room. The nurse who treated me became a friend and we prayed together. It became a very spiritual, comforting place for me."

As the tumor shrank, it unexpectedly disentangled from her major blood vessels. Surgeons removed her pancreas, gallbladder, and spleen as well as parts of her colon and liver. Amazingly, she has returned to full-time work. Receiving insulin shots and taking enzyme pills are part of her new daily regimen.

Acknowledging the wonder of her healing, she writes, "Every day is beautiful. I've learned to look at things as blessings that I used to just take for granted. The shoes I put on my feet, the hot water when I take a bath—every single aspect of my life is a blessing."

Encouraging others, Chrissy advises, "Keep looking for options and keep your faith. God took what was the scariest time in my life and turned it into a time of miracles. I am forever indebted."[a]

[a]Stacy Simons, "Pancreatic Cancer Survivor Defies Prognosis," *American Cancer Society*, October 27, 2016, www.cancer.org/latest-news/pancreatic-cancer-survivor-defies -prognosis.html.

We cultivate wonder by being with children. Children live in a world of constant wonder. Everything is novel and exciting. Brimming with vivid imaginations, children are creative, fun, and full of life. Seeing life through fresh eyes, they observe the unexpected and beautiful. Plus, they aren't shy about expressing their joy and observations. Little surprise that one of the best TV shows ever about childhood was titled *The Wonder Years*.

When I was a young dad, our eldest daughter, Laura, accused me of living a second childhood through her. Guilty as charged! I was simply thrilled floating down streams on air mattresses, eating s'mores around campfires, and improvising lyrics to made-up songs. Being near children allows their sense of wonder to infect us.

We cultivate wonder by pondering heaven. Precancer, I rarely thought about heaven. Sure, I knew it was there, but it seemed so far off. After my existential slap, however, my timespan changed radically. I now muse about it a lot. Rather than being morbid, I began to share the apostle Paul's astonishment:

> "What no eye has seen,
>> what no ear has heard,
> and what no human mind has conceived,"—
>> the things God has prepared for those who love him.[24]

Contemplating this wondrous eternal home, our fears of pain, physical limitations, and death itself are eased. The final words of Eugene Peterson, author of *The Message*, were "Let's go."[25] Likewise, as Dallas Willard succumbed to cancer, a friend observed "the unmistakable gleam of anticipation in his eyes. A childlike excitement. . . . His expectant joy was unquenchable. He knew that he was shortly to experience what he had long dreamed of and hoped for."[26]

Heaven is the ultimate wonder because our loving Father has prepared a place for each of us.[27] Those of us who have been fortunate to survive cancer are fully aware that bonus time will not last forever. Eventually, the referee's final whistle will blow. Contemplating heaven, Dietrich Bonhoeffer described himself as being "homesick" and yearning for "transformation into joyful release."[28]

THE GIFT OF WONDER

Wonder is one of God's most incredible gifts. Not only do cancer survivors experience it in extraordinary situations (like everyone else), but we also are attuned to it in the ordinary. Walking in the woods, going to church, and holding an infant all carry extra meaning for us. Humbled and grateful for our extra time on earth, epiphanies come in both quiet and dramatic settings.

Moving into liminal space and experiencing kairos moments, we cultivate God's presence through Scripture, solitude, prayer, fellowship, and worshiping communities. As we slow down, relish God's creation, and see the world through children's eyes, our sense of wonder is enhanced. Most significantly, we lean into the "hope of glory"—anticipating the day when heaven will become our permanent home.[29]

REFLECTION QUESTIONS

1. What gives you a sense of wonder?

2. What steps are you taking to cultivate wonder?

3. Reflect on excerpts from the following psalms.

Psalm 31

Praise be to the LORD,
    for he showed me the wonders of his love
    when I was in a city under siege.
In my alarm I said,
   "I am cut off from your sight!"
Yet you heard my cry for mercy
    when I called to you for help.

Love the Lord, all his faithful people!
   The Lord preserves those who are true to him,
   but the proud he pays back in full.
Be strong and take heart,
   all you who hope in the Lord.

Psalm 92

It is good to praise the Lord
   and make music to your name, O Most High,
proclaiming your love in the morning
   and your faithfulness at night. . . .
For you make me glad by your deeds, Lord;
   I sing for joy at what your hands have done.
How great are your works, Lord,
   how profound your thoughts! . . .
You have exalted my horn like that of a wild ox;
   fine oils have been poured on me.
My eyes have seen the defeat of my adversaries. . . .
The righteous will flourish like a palm tree,
   they will grow like a cedar of Lebanon;
planted in the house of the Lord,
   they will flourish in the courts of our God.
They will still bear fruit in old age,
   they will stay fresh and green,
proclaiming, "The Lord is upright;
   he is my Rock, and there is no wickedness in him."

BENEDICTION

FELLOW SURVIVORS AND CAREGIVERS,
Thank you for allowing me to travel with you. I hope that this book has been an encouragement. While each of our stories is unique, we share commonalities of faith and fear, hope and despair, joy and sadness. My goal has been to be both bluntly honest and theologically thoughtful.

Every time I look in the mirror, I see a small reminder of my medical journey. For some reason several eyelashes that fell out during chemo over my left eye never grew back. So, I have an uneven blink. One eye is normal, the other is not. The gap is symbolic of a changed life. I'm different now. Still me, but not quite the same.

My prayer is that we will become better people through our ordeals—deeper spiritually, better relationally, clearer in purpose, and stronger emotionally. In this posture of gratitude, missing eyelashes don't depress us. Rather, we see them as tokens of God's grace, reminding us both of our past rescue and future calling.

May you experience the Lord in profound ways, be surrounded by people you love, find meaningful service, and experience wonder with surprising regularity. And when your time on earth ends, may you hear our heavenly Father say, "You have lived and loved well." And may you be able to reply: "I think I stewarded bonus time pretty well. Thanks for giving it to me."

ACKNOWLEDGMENTS

S PECIAL THANKS TO MY WIFE, Mary, who served as first reader on every word of this book. Though my first draft was incredibly rough, she stayed with me through multiple rewrites. The final product reflects her efforts to make me sound less like a professor. In addition, her caregiver perspective enriches every chapter.

Thanks also to several dear friends who had a major impact on the manuscript—Scott Bryant, Gwyneth Bailey, Denise Daniels, Rudy Hernandez, Andrea Thomas, Chris Dolson, Leighton Ford, Jon Eisenberg, Carolyn Hill, Grant Hill, and Barney Ford. This has truly been a community effort.

NOTES

INTRODUCTION

[1]Anne E. K. Page and Nancy E. Adler, eds., *Cancer Care for the Whole Patient* (Washington, DC: National Academies Press, 2008), www.ncbi.nlm.nih.gov/books/NBK4011.

[2]David Scadden, *Cancerland: A Medical Memoir* (New York: St. Martin's Press, 2018), 208. See also "ACS Report: Number of US Cancer Survivors Expected to Exceed 20 Million by 2026," American Cancer Society, June 2, 2016, www.cancer.org/latest-news/report-number-of-cancer-survivors-continues-to-grow.html; "Statistics," National Cancer Institute, accessed April 30, 2019, https://cancercontrol.cancer.gov/ocs/statistics/statistics.html; and "Worldwide Cancer Statistics," Cancer Research UK, accessed April 30, 2019, www.cancerresearchuk.org/health-professional/cancer-statistics/worldwide-cancer.

1. MY STORY

[1]David Scadden, *Cancerland: A Medical Memoir* (New York: St. Martin's Press, 2018), 2.

2. GOD'S PRESENCE ON DARK DAYS

[1]Mother Teresa, quoted in Brian Kolodiejchuk, *Mother Teresa: Come Be My Light* (New York: Doubleday, 2007), 156-77.

[2]R. C. Sproul, "The Dark Night of the Soul," *Ligonier Ministries*, February 1, 2008, www.ligonier.org/learn/articles/dark-night-soul.

[3]Psalm 13:1; 28:1.

[4]Isaiah 43:1-3.

[5]Genesis 7:12; Joshua 5:6; Matthew 4:1-11.

[6]2 Corinthians 4:7.

[7]Matthew 11:28.

[8]"Persecuted Pastor's Unshakable Faith Inspires Inmates to Accept Christ," *Charisma News*, November 29, 2013, www.charismanews.com/world/41918 -persecuted-pastor-s-unshakable-faith-inspires-inmates-to-accept-christ. See also Leah Marieann Klett, "North Korean Christian Imprisoned for Her Faith Shares How God Sustained Her in Darkest Days," *Gospel Herald*, August 24, 2017, www.gospelherald.com/articles/71292/20170824/north -korean-christian-imprisoned-faith-shares-god-sustained-darkest-days.htm.

[9]John 6:68.

[10]2 Corinthians 4:16.

[11]"1 Peter 3:13-15," *Truth for Today*, accessed April 30, 2019, www.truthfortoday .co.uk/images/stories/preachit/scriptspet-cor/1_Peter_3v13-15.pdf.

[12]Deuteronomy 8:12-14.

[13]C. S. Lewis, *The Problem of Pain* (London: MacMillian, 1943), 63-64, cited in Brother Lawrence with Harold Myra, *The Practice of the Presence of God* (Grand Rapids: Discovery House, 2017), 19.

[14]Robert Robertson, *Come Thou Fount of Every Blessing*, 1757.

[15]Augustine, quoted in Kate Bowler, *Everything Happens for a Reason and Other Lies I've Loved* (New York: Random House, 2018), 122.

[16]Matthew 7:24-27.

[17]James Bryan Smith, *The Good and Beautiful God: Falling in Love with the God Jesus Knows* (Downers Grove, IL: InterVarsity Press, 2009); Richard Foster, *Celebration of Discipline: The Path to Spiritual Growth,* anniv. ed. (New York: HarperOne, 2018); Ruth Haley Barton, *Sacred Rhythms: Arranging Our Lives for Spiritual Transformation* (Downers Grove, IL: InterVarsity Press, 2006); Dallas Willard, *The Divine Conspiracy: Redis- covering Our Hidden Life in God* (New York: Harper, 1998).

[18]Hebrews 10:19-22.

3. WHY ME?

[1]Evan Sernoffsky, "Woman Shot in San Francisco's Potrero Hill," *SFGate*, July 31, 2014, www.sfgate.com/news/article/Woman-shot-in-San-Francisco -s-Potrero-Hill-5660065.php.

[2]Some philosophers distinguish between *theodicy* and *defense*. Whereas a *theodicy* tries to explain why God allows suffering, a *defense* has the more modest goal of arguing that evil is not incompatible with God's existence.

[3]Kelly Kapic, *Embodied Hope: A Theological Meditation on Pain and Suffering* (Downers Grove, IL: InterVarsity Press, 2017). See also "Gottfried Wilhelm Leibniz," *Wikipedia*, accessed May 1, 2019, https://en.wikipedia .org/wiki/Gottfried_Wilhelm_Leibniz.

[4]Voltaire, *Candide* (London: Dover Thrift Editions, 1991).

[5]Genesis 1:3-31.

[6]Alvin Plantinga, *God, Freedom and Evil* (Grand Rapids: Eerdmans, 1977), chap. 4. See also Tim Keller, *Walking with God Through Pain and Suffering* (New York: Dutton, 2013), 123.

[7]Deuteronomy 28:1-68; Leviticus 26:1-46; Galatians 6:7-9.

[8]Aimee Swartz, "Why Do Healthy Non-Smokers Get Lung Cancer?" *Atlantic*, December 3, 2013. www.theatlantic.com/health/archive/2013/12/why -do-healthy-non-smokers-get-lung-cancer/281718.

[9]Thornton Wilder, *The Bridge of San Luis Rey* (New York: Random House, 1927).

[10]Romans 8:18-22.

[11]Ecclesiastes 4:1-3.

[12]Matthew 5:45; 13:24-30.

[13]"Minnesota Reeling from Tornados," *CBS News*, March 30, 1998, www .cbsnews.com/news/minnesota-reeling-from-twisters.

[14]Émile Durkheim, *Suicide: A Study in Sociology* (New York: Free Press, 1965). See also Jerry L. Sittser, *A Grace Disguised* (Grand Rapids: Zondervan, 1995), 110.

[15]Psalm 73:5-6, 12-14.

[16]Psalm 46:2-3; 69:2, 15; 104:7-9; Zechariah 10:11. See also Michael Heiser, "Why Does the Bible Say God Battled Sea Monsters at Creation?" *Logos Talk*, October 10, 2017, https://blog.logos.com/2017/10/bible-say-god-battled -sea-monsters-creation.

[17]Simone Weil, quoted in Sittser, *Grace Disguised*, 107.

[18]Norman Anderson, quoted in Lindsay Brown, *Shining Like Stars: The Power of the Gospel in the World's Universities* (Downers Grove, IL: InterVarsity Press, 2007), 45.

[19]Michael Card, *A Better Freedom: Finding Life as Slaves of Christ* (Downers Grove, IL: InterVarsity Press, 2009).

[20]Psalm 22:1-2; 73:3-14; 59:3-4; 69:4; Job 42:7-9.

[21]Ecclesiastes 9:11-12.

[22]John 9:1-3.

[23]Colin Kruse, *John*, Tyndale New Testament Commentaries (Downers Grove, IL: InterVarsity Press, 2003), 218.

[24]Luke 13:4-5.

[25]Neal Gabler, *Walt Disney: The Triumph of American Imagination* (New York: Knopf, 2006), 623.

[26]Augustine, quoted in Craig Blaising and Carmen Hardin, *Psalms 1-50*, Ancient Christian Commentary on Scripture: Old Testament VII (Downers Grove, IL: IVP Academic, 2014), 310. See also Mark S. M. Scott, *Journey Back to God: Origen on the Problem of Evil* (Oxford: Oxford University Press, 2012).

[27]Kapic, *Embodied Hope*, 29.

[28]Daniel Simundson, quoted in Kapic, *Embodied Hope*, 31.

[29]Jeremy Weber, "Cancer Causes InterVarsity President Alec Hill to Leave Campus Ministry Early," *Christianity Today*, May 15, 2015, www.christianitytoday.com/news/2015/may/cancer-causes-intervarsity-president-alec-hill-leave-ivcf.html.

[30]Ecclesiastes 3:4.

[31]Matthew 27:46. See also Douglas Groothuis, *Walking Through Darkness: A Wife's Illness—A Philosopher's Lament* (Downers Grove, IL: InterVarsity Press, 2017), 56.

[32]Kapic, *Embodied Hope*, 36.

[33]Nancy Duff, quoted in Kapic, *Embodied Hope*, 27.

[34]Genesis 3:15; Isaiah 53:4-6, 10-12; Psalm 22:1-18.

[35]Keller, *Walking with God Through Pain and Suffering*, 121.

[36]Sittser, *Grace Disguised*, 158-59.

[37]Dietrich Bonhoeffer, *Letters and Papers from Prison* (London: SCM Press, 1967), 361.

[38]Psalm 23; Isaiah 54:5; Ezekiel 16:8; Psalm 7:11; 1 Kings 8:32.

[39]John 21:22; 2 Corinthians 12:7-9; Genesis 27:1; 48:10; Matthew 14:6-12; Acts 12:2; Hebrews 11:35-38. See also Linda Bellevue, *2 Corinthians*, IVP New Testament Commentary (Downers Grove, IL: IVP Academic, 1996), 306.

[40]Jeremiah 18:1-10.

[41]Romans 9:20.

[42]Keller, *Walking with God Through Pain and Suffering*, 45, 255.

[43]Job 40:3-5; 42:1-6.

[44]Groothuis, *Walking Through Darkness*, 41.

[45]George Washington Carver, quoted in Max Lucado, *Life to the Full* (Colorado Springs: Thomas Nelson, 2012), 11.

[46]Job 42:7.

[47]Joni Eareckson Tada, *A Place of Healing: Wrestling with the Mysteries of Suffering, Pain, and God's Sovereignty* (Colorado Springs: Cook, 2010), 15-17.

[48]Joseph Bayly, quoted in Keller, *Walking with God Through Pain and Suffering*, 245.

[49]1 Corinthians 15:42-44.

[50]Revelation 21:4.

[51]Tada, *Place of Healing*, 19.

[52]Karl Marx, *Critique of Hegel's Philosophy of Right* (1843; repr. New York: CreateSpace, 2015).

[53]Sittser, *Grace Disguised*, 90.

[54]Keller, *Walking with God Through Pain and Suffering*, 117, 121.

4. SURVIVOR'S GUILT

[1]Julie Grisham, "Guilt: A Lasting Side Effect for Cancer Survivors," *Memorial Sloan Kettering Cancer Center*, June 29, 2016, 8.

[2]Hester Hill Schnipper, "Weakening the Grip of Survivor's Guilt," *Cancer Today*, April 3, 2019, www.cancertodaymag.org/Pages/Summer2016/Weakening-the-Grip-of-Survivor-Guilt.aspx.

[3]Aaron Hass, "Survivor Guilt in Holocaust Survivors and their Children," Holocaust Teacher Resource Center, accessed May 1, 2019, www.holocaust-trc.org/a-global-perspective-on-working-with-holocaust-survivors-and-the-second-generation/survivor-guilt-in-holocaust-survivors-and-their-children. See also Phoebe Hobandec, "A Holocaust Survivor with a Burden of Guilt," *New York Times*, December 20, 2005, E5.

[4]Patricia Mazzei, "After Two Apparent Student Suicides, Parkland Grieves Again," *New York Times*, March 24, 2019, A11.

[5]Lisa Esposito, "Overcoming Cancer Survivor Guilt: Some Patients Wonder Why They Lived When Others Died," *US News and World Report*, October 28, 2016, https://health.usnews.com/wellness/articles/2016-10-28/overcoming-cancer-survivor-guilt. See also Tara Perloff, Megan Johnson Shen, Maureen Rigney, and Jennifer King, "Survivor

Guilt: The Secret Burden of Cancer Survivorship," *Journal of Clinical Oncology* 34, no. 3 (January 2016): 192.

[6]Laurie Wertich, "Moving Beyond Survivor Guilt," *Thrive Magazine*, May 9, 2018, www.cancercompass.com/cancer-news/article/moving-beyond -survivor-guilt.

[7]Gordon Thomas and Max Morgan-Witts, *Voyage of the Damned* (New York: Ballantine Books, 1974).

[8]Grisham, "Guilt," 2, 5.

[9]Pam Parker, "I Survived Cancer. So Why Was I So Sad?" *Washington Post*, October 24, 2017, www.washingtonpost.com/news/posteverything /wp/2017/10/24/i-survived-cancer-so-why-was-i-so-sad/?utm_term =.fcc6352dc3b6.

[10]Radiant Racheli, "Survivor's Guilt After Ovarian Cancer," *Lymphoma News Today*, January 4, 2018, 3. See also Matthew Tull, "An Overview of Post-Traumatic Stress Disorder (PTSD)," *Very Well Mind*, April 30, 2018, www.verywellmind.com/an-overview-of-ptsd-2797638.

[11]Jamie Hutchings, "Depression and Survivor's Guilt After Leukemia," *Children's Cancer Research Fund*, June 14, 2016, https://childrenscancer.org /depression-and-survivors-guilt-after-leukemia.

[12]Judith Guest, *Ordinary People* (London: Penguin Books, 1982).

[13]"Survivor's Guilt," *Stupid Cancer Community*, November 2011.

[14]Jerry L. Sittser, *A Grace Disguised* (Grand Rapids: Zondervan, 1995), 42.

[15]Angela Long, "Survivor's Guilt—Let Me Count the Ways," *Oncology Nurse* 7, no. 4 (July-August 2014), http://jhoponline.com/ton-issue -archive/2014-issues/july-august-vol-7-no-4/16184-survivor-s-guilt -let-me-count-the-ways.

[16]Luke 12:48; 6:38 NRSV.

[17]Brad Zebrack, "Reframing the Picture," University of Michigan Rogel Cancer Center, May 10, 2018.

[18]Michael Levin, quoted in Esposito, "Overcoming Cancer Survivor's Guilt," 1-2.

[19]"Dealing with 'Survivor Guilt' After Cancer," Facing Cancer Together, May 10, 2018, at https://facingcancertogether.witf.org/living-with-cancer /dealing-with-survivor-guilt-after-cancer-61112.

[20]2 Corinthians 1:3-4, 6-7.

[21]"Peer Support Groups," Trauma Survivors Network, accessed May 1, 2019, www.traumasurvivorsnetwork.org/pages/peer-support-groups.

5. THE ILLUSION OF CONTROL

[1]Portions of this chapter first appeared in Alec Hill, "How Cancer Shattered My Illusion of Control," *Christianity Today*, December 4, 2017, www .christianitytoday.com/ct/2017/december-web-only/how-cancer-shattered -my-illusion-of-control.html. See "Illusion of Control," *Science Daily*, June 18, 2018, www.sciencedaily.com/terms/illusion_of_control.htm. See also Fred Ayeroff and Robert P. Abelson, "ESP and ESB: Belief in Personal Success at Mental Telepathy," *Journal of Personality and Social Psychology* 34 (1976): 240-47; and Francesca Gino, Zachariah Sharek, and Don Moore, "Keeping the Illusion of Control Under Control: Ceilings, Floors, and Imperfect Calibration," *Organizational Behavior and Human Decision Processes* 114, no. 2 (2011): 104-14.

[2]Michael Luo, "For Exercise in New York Futility, Push Button," *New York Times*, February 27, 2004, A1. See also Tim Dingle, "Illusion of Control in Business," Linked In, November 18, 2014, www.linkedin.com/pulse /20141118112121-88435916-illusion-of-control-in-business.

[3]William Ernest Henley, *Invictus*, 1888.

[4]Henri Nouwen, *Turn My Mourning into Dancing: Finding Hope in Hard Times* (Nashville: Thomas Nelson, 2001), 28.

[5]Tim Keller, *Walking with God Through Pain and Suffering* (New York: Dutton, 2013), 190.

[6]James 4:13-15.

[7]Dingle, "Illusion of Control in Business," 1.

[8]Max Lucado, *Anxious for Nothing: Finding Calm in a Chaotic World* (Nashville: Thomas Nelson, 2017), 148.

[9]Lucado, *Anxious for Nothing*, 95.

[10]Amy Morin, "Seven Signs of a Control Freak," *Psychology Today*, May 28, 2017, www.psychologytoday.com/us/blog/what-mentally-strong-people -dont-do/201705/7-signs-control-freak.

[11]Carl Anthony, "Rich Celebrity First Mom: Franklin Roosevelt's Dominant Mother Sara," Carl Anthony Online (blog), May 9, 2015, https://carl anthonyonline.com/2015/05/09/rich-celebrity-mom-franklin-roosevelts -dominant-mother-sara.

[12]Traci Newsom, "How to Cope with Loss of Control as a Cancer Patient," University of Texas MD Anderson Cancer Center, May 18, 2015, www .mdanderson.org/publications/cancerwise/how-to-cope-with-loss-of -control-as-a-cancer-patient.h00-158987445.html.

[13]Bridgette Ross, "Dealing with Control Issues," *Ross Psychology*, May 4, 2016, http://rosspsychology.com/blog/dealing-with-control-issues-by -redirecting-efforts-to-control-your-world.

[14]Dena Rosenbloom, Mary Beth Williams, and Barbara Watkins, *Life After Trauma* (New York: Guilford Press, 1999), 183-95.

[15]Genesis 1:27-30.

[16]Matthew 5:3.

[17]Matthew 6:25-27, 32-34.

[18]John Stott, *The Message of the Sermon on the Mount* (Downers Grove, IL: InterVarsity Press, 1978), 167.

[19]Jeremy Webber, "Cancer Causes InterVarsity President Alec Hill to Leave Campus Ministry Early," *Christianity Today*, May 15, 2015, www.christianity today.com/news/2015/may/cancer-causes-intervarsity-president-alec-hill -leave-ivcf.html.

[20]Lucado, *Anxious for Nothing*, 32.

[21]Philippians 4:4, 6, 11.

[22]Romans 8:35, 38.

[23]2 Corinthians 4:16-18.

[24]Lucado, *Anxious for Nothing*, 21.

[25]Steve Hayner and Sharol Hayner, *Joy in the Journey: Finding Abun- dance in the Shadow of Death* (Downers Grove, IL: InterVarsity Press, 2015), 89.

[26]David Desteno, "The Only Way to Keep Your Resolutions," *New York Times*, December 29, 2017, SR1. See also David Desteno, *Emotional Success: The Power of Gratitude, Compassion, and Pride* (New York: Houghton Mifflin Harcourt, 2018).

[27]Hebrews 4:9.

[28]Abraham Heschel, *The Sabbath* (New York: Farrar, Straus and Giroux, 1951), 23, 29, 30, 74, 75.

[29]Nouwen, *Turn My Mourning into Dancing*, 27.

6. DEPENDING ON OTHERS

[1]Rod Serling, "Time Enough at Last," *The Twilight Zone*, John Brahm, di- rector, airdate November 20, 1959.

[2]John Donne, *No Man Is an Island*, 1624.

[3]Brené Brown, quoted in Emma Seppala, "Connect to Thrive," *Psychology Today*, August 26, 2012, www.psychologytoday.com/us/blog/feeling-it /201208/connect-thrive.

[4]Matt Sliger, "The Illusion of Control," January 23, 2018, *Founders Ministry*, https://founders.org/2018/01/23/the-illusion-of-control.

[5]Paul Kalanithi, *When Breath Becomes Air* (New York: Random House, 2016), 217-18.

[6]Joni Eareckson Tada, *A Place of Healing: Wrestling with the Mysteries of Suffering, Pain, and God's Sovereignty* (Colorado Springs: Cook, 2010), 30-32.

[7]Mark 2:1-12.

[8]Seppala, "Connect to Thrive," 2.

[9]Dean Ornish, *Love & Survival: The Scientific Basis for the Healing Power of Intimacy* (New York: HarperCollins, 1998), 3, 14.

[10]Pat Magrath, "Oncology Nurses Are in High Demand," *Diversity Nursing*, February 13, 2017, http://blog.diversitynursing.com/blog/oncology-nurses -are-in-high-demand.

[11]Parts of this and the next three paragraphs first appeared in Alec Hill, "Eighty-Seven Days of Infusing Hope," *Journal of Christian Nursing* 35, no. 3 (July 2018): 201, https://insights.ovid.com/crossref?an=00005217 -201807000-00019.

[12]David Scadden, *Cancerland: A Medical Memoir* (New York: St. Martin's Press, 2018), 59.

[13]Proverbs 15:30 NLT.

[14]Luke 10:33-34.

[15]Angelina Gibson, "Pope Francis Calls Nurses, 'Experts in Humanity,'" *Nurse.org*, March 6, 2018, https://nurse.org/articles/pope-francis-thanks -nurses-remembers-nun.

[16]Margaret Josephson Rinck, "Becoming a Healing Community," *Christianity Today*, August 31, 2000, www.christianitytoday.com/ct/2000 /augustweb-only/40.0c.html.

[17]Jerry L. Sittser, *A Grace Disguised* (Grand Rapids: Zondervan, 1995), 171.

[18]Siddhartha Mukherjee, *The Emperor of All Maladies: A Biography of Cancer* (New York: Scribner, 2010), 420-22.

[19]Mukherjee, *Emperor of All Maladies*, 309.

[20]Elisa Criado, "Cancer Patients Often Face Relationship Problems," *Independent*, August 27, 2014, www.independent.co.uk/life-style/health-and -families/cancer-patients-often-face-relationship-problems-9692572.

html. See also "Coping with Anger," Cancer.net, March 2019, www.cancer
.net/coping-with-cancer/managing-emotions/coping-with-anger.

[21] Frances Goodhart and Lucy Atkins, "The Downside of Beating Cancer,"
Daily Mail, June 14, 2011, www.dailymail.co.uk/health/article-2003214
/Cancer-survivors-Depression-exhaustion-anger-downside-beating-disease
.html. See also "Cancer Survivors: Managing Your Emotions After Cancer
Treatment," Mayo Clinic, accessed May 2, 2019, www.mayoclinic.org
/diseases-conditions/cancer/in-depth/cancer-survivor/art-20047129; and
"Your Emotions After Treatment," Dana-Farber Cancer Institute, accessed
May 2, 2019, www.dana-farber.org/for-patients-and-families/for-survivors
/caring-for-yourself-after-cancer/your-emotions-after-treatment.

[22] "Dependent Personality Disorder," *Psychology Today*, accessed May 2,
2019, www.psychologytoday.com/us/conditions/dependent-personality
-disorder.

[23] Lisa Fayed, "Learning to Cope During Your Partner's Cancer Treatment,"
Very Well Health, August 23, 2018, www.verywellhealth.com/when
-cancer-affects-your-marriage-513974.

[24] Brenda Avadian, "Top Mistakes New Caregivers Make," *U.S. News and
World Report*, August 19, 2016, https://health.usnews.com/health-news
/patient-advice/articles/2016-08-19/top-mistakes-new-caregivers-make.

[25] "If You're About to Become a Cancer Caregiver," American Cancer Society,
June 6, 2016, www.cancer.org/treatment/caregivers/if-youre-about-to
-become-a-cancer-caregiver.html.

[26] Meda Freeman, "Caregivers' Stress Leads to Unhealthy Habits," *California
Health Report*, October 2, 2011, www.calhealthreport.org/2011/10/02
/caregivers-stress-leads-to-unhealthy-habits.

[27] "Men Leave: Separation and Divorce Far More Common When the Wife
Is the Patient," *Science Daily*, November 10, 2009, www.sciencedaily.com
/releases/2009/11/091110105401.htm. See also Tara Parker-Pope, "Divorce
Risk Higher When Wife Gets Sick," *New York Times*, November 12, 2009,
https://well.blogs.nytimes.com/2009/11/12/men-more-likely-to-leave
-spouse-with-cancer.

[28] Youngmee Kim, Frank Baker, and Rachel Spillers, "Cancer Caregivers'
Quality of Life: Effects of Gender, Relationship, and Appraisal," *Journal
of Pain and Symptom Management* 34 (2007): 298-302.

[29] Meredith Bryan, "When Spouse Gets Sick, Who Leaves?" *CNN*, July 21,
2011, www.cnn.com/2011/LIVING/07/21/sick.couples.o.

[30]Bryan, "When Spouse Gets Sick, Who Leaves?"

7. IDENTITY

[1]Cynthia Mathieson and Henderikus Stam, "Renegotiating Identity: Cancer Narratives," *Sociology of Health & Illness* 17, no. 3 (1995): 283-306. See also Brad Zebrack, "Cancer Survivor Identity and Quality of Life," *Cancer Practice* 8 (September 2000): 238-42.

[2]Portions of this chapter first appeared in Alec Hill, "My New Life as a Chimera: Living with Two Sets of DNA," *Christianity Today*, March 3, 2016. See also "Chimerism-Testing," Seattle Cancer Care Alliance, October 20, 2018, www .seattlecca.org/healthcare-professionals/clinical-labs/clinical -immunogenetics-laboratory/chimerism-testing; and "Chimera (mythology)," *New World Encyclopedia*, October 20, 2018, www.newworldencyclopedia.org /entry/Chimera_(mythology).

[3]Crystal Park, Ianita Zlateva, and Thomas Blank, "Self-identity After Cancer: Survivor, Victim, Patient, and Person with Cancer," *Journal of General Internal Medicine* 24, sup. 2 (November 2009): 430-35.

[4]Ed Mitchell, "The Sick Role," *National Health Service New England*, September 30, 2013, www.england.nhs.uk/blog/ed-mitchell-2. See also Sze Yan Cheung and Paul Delfabbro, "Are You a Cancer Survivor? A Review on Cancer Identity," *Journal of Cancer Survivorship* 10, no. 4 (August 2016): 759-71.

[5]Stacy Simon, "Survivors: Words of Inspiration," American Cancer Society, May 28, 2013, www.cancer.org/latest-news/survivors-words-of-inspiration .html.

[6]Mathieson and Stam, "Renegotiating Identity," 294.

[7]2 Corinthians 4:7-9. See also Michael Bird, "A Christian View of Human Identity," *Patheos*, October 26, 2018, www.patheos.com/blogs/euangelion /2018/10/a-christian-view-of-human-identity.

[8]Sara Hardy, Kevin Krull, Jeffrey Wefel, and Michelle Janelsins, "Cognitive Changes in Cancer Survivors," *American Society of Clinical Oncology Educational Book* 38 (2018): 795-806. See also Brad Zebrack, "Cancer Survivor Identity and Quality of Life," *Cancer Practice* 8 (September 2000): 241.

[9]Quote provided by a Seattle Cancer Care Alliance nurse.

[10]1 Corinthians 15:35-49.

[11]"Your Emotions After Treatment," Dana Farber Cancer Institute, accessed May 3, 2019, www.dana-farber.org/for-patients-and-families/for-survivors/caring-for-yourself-after-cancer/your-emotions-after-treatment. See also Ros Taylor, "Relationships, Sex and Intimacy," Target Ovarian Cancer, April 8, 2019, www.targetovariancancer.org.uk/information-and-support/my-ovarian-cancer-incurable/relationships-sex-and-intimacy.

[12]Sema Koçan and Ayla Gürsoy, "Body Image of Women with Breast Cancer After Mastectomy: A Qualitative Research," *Journal of Breast Cancer* 12, no. 4 (October 2016): 145-50.

[13]Clara Nan-hi Lee, Michael Pignone, and Allison Deal, "Accuracy of Predictions of Patients with Breast Cancer of Future Well-being After Immediate Breast Reconstruction," *JAMA Surgery* 4 (2018): 153.

[14]Zebrack, "Cancer Survivor Identity and Quality of Life," 243.

[15]PJ Hamel, "The Line in the Sand: When a Friend Disappears After Your Cancer Diagnosis," Health Central, March 14, 2018, www.healthcentral.com/article/why-friends-may-disappear-after-your-cancer-diagnosis.

[16]Katie Taylor, "7 Reasons Why Friends Might Abandon You During Cancer and How to Cope," *TheBreastCancerSite.com* (blog), March 28, 2019, https://blog.thebreastcancersite.greatergood.com/cancer-abandonment. See also Harriet Brown, "Coping with Crises Close to Someone Else's Heart," *New York Times*, August 16, 2010, D5.

[17]Anne Moyer, "Cancer and Stigma," *Psychology Today*, August 1, 2017, www.psychologytoday.com/us/blog/beyond-treatment/201708/cancer-and-stigma.

[18]V. Vaughn-Sandler, C. Sherman, A. Aronsohn, and M. Volk, "Consequences of Perceived Stigma Among Patients with Cirrhosis," *Digestive Diseases and Science* 59, no. 3 (March 2014): 681-86. See also R. Shabanloei, H. Ebrahimi, F. Ahmadi, E. Mohammadi, and R. Dolatkhah, "Stigma in Cirrhotic Patients: A Qualitative Study," *Gastroentoral Nursing* 39, no. 3 (May-June 2016): 216-26.

[19]Anna Wagstaff, "Stigma: Breaking the Vicious Cycle," *Cancerworld*, July 1, 2013, https://cancerworld.net/patient-voice/stigma-breaking-the-vicious-cycle.

[20]Tim Keller, *Counterfeit Gods* (New York: Riverhead, 2009), xvi.

[21]Elaine Shattner, "Get Cancer. Lose Your Job?" *Medical Lessons*, March 26, 2019, www.medicallessons.net/category/breast. See also Reshma Jagsi et al., "Impact of Adjuvant Chemotherapy on Long-Term Employment of

Survivors of Early-Stage Breast Cancer," *Cancer* 120, no. 12 (June 2014): 1854-62; and "One-Fifth of Cancer Patients Face Work Discrimination," BBC News, November 7, 2016, www.bbc.com/news/health-37861712.

[22]Steve Hayner and Sharol Hayner, *Joy in the Journey: Finding Abundance in the Shadow of Death* (Downers Grove, IL: InterVarsity Press, 2015), 89.

[23]Ephesians 2:10; 2 Corinthians 3:17-18 NLT.

[24]Dietrich Bonhoeffer, "Who Am I?" DBonhoeffer.org, April 9, 2019, www .dbonhoeffer.org/who-was-db2.htm.

PART Three: LIVING IN BONUS TIME

[1]Eight died and came back to life: (1) the widow of Zarephath's son (1 Kings 17:17-24); (2) the Shunamite's son (2 Kings 4:20-37); (3) a man tossed into Elisha's tomb (2 Kings 13:21); (4) a widow's son (Luke 7:11-17); (5) Jairus's daughter (Mark 5:35-43); (6) Lazarus (John 11:1-44); (7) Tabitha (Acts 9:36-41); and (8) Eutychus (Acts 20:7-12). In addition, (9) Hezekiah's life was extended fifteen years (2 Kings 20:6).

[2]John 12:10-11.

[3]Lazarus continues to fascinate. A wide range of artists—including Bob Dylan, Chinua Achebe (*Things Fall Apart*), Vincent van Gogh, Donald Glover (film director), and David Bowie—have all used his name in titles of their works.

8. SURVIVOR'S GROWTH

[1]David Kushner, "Can Trauma Help You Grow?" *New Yorker*, March 15, 2016, www.newyorker.com/tech/annals-of-technology/can-trauma-help -you-grow.

[2]Ryan Denney, Jamie Aten, and Kari Leavell, "Post Traumatic Growth: A Phenomenological Study of Cancer Patients," *Journal of Mental Health, Religion, and Culture* 14, no. 4 (2011): 311-22.

[3]Eric Maisel, quoted in Tim Keller, *Walking with God Through Pain and Suffering* (New York: Dutton, 2013), 188-89.

[4]Job 17:9 NLT.

[5]Richard Tedeschi and James Calhoun, quoted in Jim Rendon, "Post-Traumatic Stress's Surprisingly Positive Flip Side," *New York Times Magazine*, March 22, 2012, MM38.

[6]James 1:2-4.

[7]Isaiah 38:1-22.

[8]They include (1) change priorities, (2) establish a new life pathway, (3) do better things, (4) develop new interests, (5) value life more, (6) appreciate each day, (7) put more effort into relationships, (8) be more compassionate, (9) express emotions, (10) appreciate others, (11) need others, (12) handle difficulties, (13) have stronger religious faith, (14) understand spiritual matters, (15) accept new self, (16) pursue new opportunities, (17) change things, (18) exercise self-reliance, (19) count on others, (20) be stronger, (21) be closer to others. See Kanako Taku, Arnie Cann, Lawrence Calhoun, and Richard Tedeschi, "The Factor Structure of the Posttraumatic Growth Inventory: A Comparison of Five Models Using Confirmatory Factor Analysis," *Journal of Traumatic Stress* 21, no. 2 (April 2008): 158-64.

[9]Angela Duckworth, *Grit: The Power of Passion and Perseverance* (New York: Scribner, 2016), 55. See also Margaret Perlis, "5 Characteristics of Grit—How Many Do You Have?" *Forbes*, October 29, 2013, www.forbes .com/sites/margaretperlis/2013/10/29/5-characteristics-of-grit-what -it-is-why-you-need-it-and-do-you-have-it/#66263cd74f7b.

[10]Meg Jay, *Supernormal: The Untold Stories of Adversity and Resilience* (New York: Hachette, 2017), 8.

[11]Jim Rendon, *Upside: The New Science of Post-Traumatic Growth* (New York: Touchstone, 2015), xv.

[12]Romans 5:3-4.

[13]John Stott, *Romans: God's Good News for the World* (Downers Grove, IL: InterVarsity Press, 1994), 142.

[14]Ed Smith, "The Voodoo Cult of Positive Thinking: Lessons from Lance Armstrong's Disgrace," *New Statesman*, September 6, 2012, www.newstatesman .com/culture/books/2012/09/voodoo-cult-positive-thinking. See also Ephesians 2:4-10.

[15]Rendon, *Upside*, 178, 183-84.

[16]Richard Tedeschi and Lawrence Calhoun, "Posttraumatic Growth: Conceptual Foundations and Empirical Evidence," *Psychological Inquiry* 15, no. 1 (2004): 1-18.

[17]Gabriele Prati and Luca Pietrantoni, cited in Rendon, *Upside*, 148.

[18]Annick Shaw, Stephen Joseph, S. Joseph, and Alex Linley, "Religion, Spirituality, and Post-Traumatic Growth: A Systematic Review," *Mental Health, Religion & Culture* 8, no. 1 (2004): 1-11. See also Amanda Gesselman et al., "Spirituality, Emotional Distress, and Post-Traumatic Growth in Breast

Cancer Survivors and Their Partners," *Northwestern University*, October 1, 2017, www.scholars.northwestern.edu/en/publications/spirituality -emotional-distress-and-post-traumatic-growth-in-brea; Shelley Wiechman Askay and Gina Magyar-Russell, "Post-Traumatic Growth and Spirituality in Burn Recovery," *International Review of Psychiatry* 21 (2009): 570-79; Justin O'Rourke, Benjamin Tallman, and Elizabeth Altmaier, "Measuring Post-Traumatic Changes in Spirituality/Religiosity," *Mental Health, Religion & Culture* 11, no. 7 (2008): 719-28; Irene Harris et al., "Coping Functions of Prayer and Posttraumatic Growth," *International Journal for the Psychology of Religion* 20 (2010): 26-38.

[19]Denney, Aten, and Leavell, "Post Traumatic Growth," 16.

[20]Joanna Mercuri, "Pastoral Counselor Explores Link Between Spirituality and Post-Traumatic Growth," *Fordham News*, July 16, 2012, https://news .fordham.edu/inside-fordham-category/pastoral-counselor -explores-link-between-spirituality-and-post-traumatic-growth.

[21]Rendon, *Upside*, 12-15, 236.

[22]Ayse Nuray Karanci, quoted in Rendon, *Upside*, 165.

[23]Richard Tedeshi and Lawrence Calhoun, "The Posttraumatic Growth Inventory: Measuring the Positive Legacy of Trauma," *Journal of Traumatic Stress* 9, no. 3 (July 1996): 455-71. See also John Piper, "The Fruit of Hope: Boldness," Desiring God, July 20, 1986, www.desiringgod.org /messages/the-fruit-of-hope-boldness.

[24]Pam Parker, "I Survived Cancer. Why Was I So Sad?" *Washington Post*, October 24, 2017, www.newsday.com/opinion/commentary/i-survived -cancer-why-was-i-so-sad-1.14651882.

[25]Juan Ortega and Ihosvani Rodriguez, "Woman, 66, Tackles Robber, Credits Her Cancer for Giving Her Bravery," *Sun Sentinel*, April 1, 2011, www.sun-sentinel.com/news/fl-xpm-2011-04-01-fl-oakland-park-bank -robbery-20110401-story.html.

[26]Joshua 1:6-16; Luke 19:11-26; 2 Corinthians 3:12; 2 Timothy 1:7.

[27]Jerry Sittser, *A Grace Disguised: How the Soul Grows through Loss* (Grand Rapids: Zondervan, 2004), 45.

9. CLARITY OF PURPOSE

[1]Dhruv Khullar, "Finding Purpose for a Good Life. But Also a Healthy One," *New York Times*, January 1, 2018, www.nytimes.com/2018/01/01

/upshot/finding-purpose-for-a-good-life-but-also-a-healthy-one.html. See also Ryan Denney, Jamie Aten, and Kari Leavell, "Posttraumatic Spiritual Growth: A Phenomenological Study of Cancer," *Mental Health, Religion & Culture* 14 (2011), https://aquila.usm.edu/cgi/viewcontent.cgi?a rticle=2084&context=dissertations.

²Yael Ridberg, "On Eagle's Wings—A Rabbi Confronts Her Cancer Diagnosis During the High Holidays," Jewish Reconstructionist Communities, accessed May 7, 2019, http://archive.jewishrecon.org/resource/eagles -wings%E2%80%94-rabbi-confronts-her-cancer-diagnosis-during -high-holidays.

³David Scadden, *Cancerland: A Medical Memoir* (New York: St. Martin's Press, 2018), 83.

⁴Patrick Hill, "Having a Sense of Purpose May Add Years to Your Life," *Association for Psychological Science*, May 12, 2014, www.psychologicalscience .org/news/releases/having-a-sense-of-purpose-in-life-may-add-years-to -your-life.html. See also Khullar, "Finding Purpose for a Good Life."

⁵Patti Neighmond, "People Who Feel They Have a Purpose in Life Live Longer," NPR Health News, July 28, 2014, www.npr.org/sections/health -shots/2014/07/28/334447274/people-who-feel-they-have-a-purpose-in -life-live-longer.

⁶Atul Gawande, *Being Mortal: Medicine and What Matters at the End* (New York: Holt, 2014), 125.

⁷Emily Espahani Smith, "How to Find Meaning in the Face of Death," *Atlantic*, March 2, 2017, www.theatlantic.com/health/archive/2017/03 /power-of-meaning/518196.

⁸Paul Kalanithi, *When Breath Becomes Air* (New York: Random House, 2016), 214.

⁹Robert Fulghum, quoted in Michael Yaconeli, *Dangerous Wonder: The Adventure of Childlike Faith* (Colorado Springs: NavPress, 1998), 95.

¹⁰Suleika Jaouad, "Lost in Transition After Cancer," *New York Times*, March 16, 2015, D6.

¹¹Brother Lawrence with Harold Myra, *The Practice of the Presence of God* (Grand Rapids: Discovery House, 2017), 35.

¹²1 Corinthians 6:19-20.

¹³Alec Hill, "Inside My Slavery," *Christianity Today*, July-August 2014, 76.

¹⁴Galatians 2:20.

¹⁵Mike Riccardi, "Slaves of Christ," *The Cripplegate*, September 14, 2012,

http://thecripplegate.com/slaves-of-christ.

[16]Frederich Buechner, *Wishful Thinking: A Seeker's ABC* (New York: Harper, 1993), 95.

[17]Anna Moore, "Life After Breast Cancer: Three Survivors' Stories," *Telegraph*, November 8, 2012, www.telegraph.co.uk/lifestyle/9615701/Life-after-breast-cancer-three-survivors-stories.html.

[18]Valerie Yates, quoted in Moore, "Life After Breast Cancer."

[19]Roy Sessions, "Finding New Purpose After Enduring the Cancer Experience," *Psychology Today*, January 19, 2014, www.psychologytoday.com/us/blog/the-cancer-experience/201401/finding-new-purpose-after-enduring-the-cancer-experience.

[20]Leighton Ford, *The Attentive Life: Discerning God's Presence in All Things* (Downers Grove, IL: InterVarsity Press, 2008), 13.

[21]Tiffany Shlain, "Tech's Best Feature: The Off Switch," *Harvard Business Review*, March 1, 2013. https://hbr.org/2013/03/techs-best-feature-the-off-swi.

10. REDEEMING TIME

[1]Greek rendering of Ephesians 5:15-16.

[2]Jennie Dear, "What It's Like to Learn You're Going to Die," *Atlantic*, November 2, 2017, www.theatlantic.com/health/archive/2017/11/the-existential-slap/544790.

[3]Sarah Sullivan-Singh, Annette Stanton, and Carissa Low, "Living with Limited Time: Socioemotional Selectivity Theory in the Context of Health Adversity," *Journal of Personality and Social Psychology* 108, no. 6 (June 2015): 900-16.

[4]Atul Gawande, *Being Mortal: Medicine and What Matters at the End* (New York: Holt, 2014), 97.

[5]Sullivan-Singh, Stanton, and Low, "Living with Limited Time," 913.

[6]Psalm 90:12.

[7]Benjamin Franklin, "Poor Richard 1746," Founders Online, accessed May 7, 2019, https://founders.archives.gov/documents/Franklin/01-03-02-0025.

[8]Billy Graham, quoted in Brother Lawrence with Harold Myra, *The Practice of the Presence of God* (Grand Rapids: Discovery House, 2017), 113.

[9]Paul Kalanithi, *When Breath Becomes Air* (New York: Random House, 2016), 161-62.

[10]Henri Nouwen, *Turn My Mourning into Dancing: Finding Hope in Hard Times* (Nashville: Thomas Nelson, 2001), 54. See also Jim Erwin, "Psalm 90:1-12 Time Management," *Patheos*, January 5, 2014, www.patheos .com/blogs/jimerwin/2014/01/05/psalm-901-12-time-management.

[11]"Psalm 90:12," Bible Hub, accessed May 7, 2019, http://biblehub.com /commentaries/hastings/psalms/90-12.htm.

[12]Sue Bourne, "What Would You do if You Had Only 12 Months to Live?" *Telegraph*, May 17, 2017, www.telegraph.co.uk/women/life/would-do-had -12-months-live-learned-filming-dying.

[13]Shannon Miller, quoted in Stacy Simon, "Lessons from the Olympics Help Shannon Miller Through Ovarian Cancer Treatment," American Cancer Society, September 2, 2016, www.cancer.org/latest-news/lessons -from-the-olympics-help-shannon-miller-through-ovarian-cancer -treatment.html.

[14]Gawande, *Being Mortal*, 97.

[15]Kate Bowler, *Everything Happens for a Reason and Other Lies I've Loved* (New York: Random House, 2018), 165.

[16]Liz Mineo, "Good Genes are Nice, But Joy Is Better," *Harvard Gazette*, April 11, 2017, https://news.harvard.edu/gazette/story/2017/04/over -nearly-80-years-harvard-study-has-been-showing-how-to-live-a -healthy-and-happy-life.

[17]Tim Nichols and Craig Wiseman, "Live Like You Were Dying," Curb Records, 2004.

[18]John Claypool, quoted in Michael Yaconelli, *Dangerous Wonder: The Adventure of Childlike Faith* (Colorado Springs: NavPress, 2003), 92-93.

[19]Hubert Humphrey, quoted in Steve Brown, "What Would You Do Differently If This Were Your Last Year?" Crosswalk.com, August 20, 2001, www .crosswalk.com/faith/spiritual-life/what-would-you-do-differently-if -this-were-your-last-year-755532.html.

[20]Malachy McCourt, quoted in Amy Rees Anderson, "Resentment Is Like Taking Poison and Waiting for the Other Person to Die," *Forbes*, April 7, 2015, www.forbes.com/sites/amyanderson/2015/04/07/resentment-is -like-taking-poison-and-waiting-for-the-other-person-to-die/#126 e034b446c.

[21]Matthew 5:43-48.

[22]Steve Jobs, "You've Got to Find What You Love," *Stanford News*, June 14, 2005, https://news.stanford.edu/2005/06/14/jobs-061505.

[23]Laura Nott, "Is Watching Too Much TV Making You Depressed? Studies Say It Can," *Elements: Behavioral Health,* July 12, 2013, www.promises behavioralhealth.com/addiction-recovery-blog/is-watching-too-much -tv-making-you-depressed. See also Olinka Koster, "Why Using a Computer Can Cause Depression," *Daily Mail,* reviewed May 17, 2019, www .dailymail.co.uk/health/article-153281/Why-using-cause-depression.html.

[24]Nouwen, *Turn My Mourning into Dancing,* 67.

[25]Bowler, *Everything Happens for a Reason,* 144.

[26]Tim Keller, *Walking with God Through Pain and Suffering* (New York: Dutton, 2013), 192.

11. WONDER

[1]Jonathan Haidt and Dacher Keltner, "Approaching Awe, a Moral, Spiritual and Aesthetic Emotion," *Journal of Cognition and Emotion* 17 (2003): 297-300.

[2]Andrew Tix, "Overwhelmed by Greatness: The Psychological Significance of Awe in Christian Experience and Formation," *Biola University Center for Christian Thought,* October 26, 2015, https://cct.biola.edu/over whelmed-greatness-psychological-significance-awe-christian-experience -and-formation.

[3]Shaun Gallagher et al., *A Neurophenomenology of Awe and Wonder: Towards a Non-Reductionist Cognitive Science* (London: Palgrave Mac-Millan, 2015).

[4]Haidt and Keltner, "Approaching Awe," 302, 309.

[5]Abraham Maslow, quoted in Haidt and Keltner, "Approaching Awe," 302.

[6]Matthew 17:6; Mark 6:8; Acts 9:1-30.

[7]C. S. Lewis, *The Chronicles of Narnia* (London: Geoffrey Bles, 1956).

[8]Kate Bowler, *Everything Happens for a Reason and Other Lies I've Loved* (New York: Random House, 2018), 120.

[9]Jeffrey Long, "Stories of God's Love Common Among Those Who Almost Die," *Washington Post,* June 29, 2016, www.washingtonpost.com/news/acts -of-faith/wp/2016/06/29/people-who-had-near-death-experiences -consistently-report-one-thing-gods-love. See also Helen Thompson, "Near-Death Experiences Are Overwhelmingly Peaceful," *New Science,* June 26, 2014, www.newscientist.com/article/dn25794-near-death-experiences-are -overwhelmingly-peaceful.

[10]Jim Rendon, "Post-Traumatic Stress's Surprisingly Positive Flip Side," *New York Times,* March 22, 2012, MM38.

[11]Margaret Feinberg, *Wonderstruck: Awaken to the Nearness of God* (Franklin, TN: Worthy Publishing, 2012).

[12]Psalm 119:129 ESV.

[13]Tanya Luhrmann, quoted by Tix, "Overwhelmed by Greatness," 8.

[14]Michael Card, *Mark: The Gospel of Passion* (Downers Grove, IL: InterVarsity Press, 2012), 5.

[15]Jesse Hill, "Wonder and Worship," Pilpott Memorial Church, October 20, 2017, www.acommunityofgrace.org/blog/2017/10/20/wonder-and-worship.

[16]Leighton Ford, *The Attentive Life: Discerning God's Presence in All Things* (Downers Grove, IL: InterVarsity Press, 2008), 109.

[17]Matthew 4:4.

[18]Greg McKeown, *Essentialism* (New York: Random House, 2014), 4.

[19]Job 37:14; Isaiah 29:9.

[20]Shannon Harvey, "The Amazing Health Benefits of Awe and Wonder," Connection, June 18, 2015, https://theconnection.tv/the-amazing-health-benefits-of-awe-and-wonder.

[21]Ford, *Attentive Life*, 38, 109.

[22]Margaret Feinberg, "Don't Lose the Wonder: How I Rediscovered the Splendor of Being God's Own," *Christianity Today's Leadership Journal,* spring 2013, 87.

[23]Barbara Frederickson, cited by Tix, "Overwhelmed by Greatness," 9.

[24]1 Corinthians 2:9.

[25]Emily McFarlan Miller, "Eugene Peterson, Author of 'The Message' and Pastor to Other Pastors, Dies at Age 85," Religion News Service, October 22, 2018, https://religionnews.com/2018/10/22/eugene-peterson-obit-died-at-85-the-message.

[26]Gary Black, *Preparing for Heaven: What Dallas Willard Taught Me About Living, Dying and Eternal Life* (New York: Harper One, 2015), xxii.

[27]John 14:1-4.

[28]Eric Metaxas, *Bonhoeffer: Pastor, Martyr, Prophet, Spy* (Nashville: Thomas Nelson, 2010), 517.

[29]Colossians 1:27.

RECOMMENDED BOOKS

1. MY STORY

Scadden, David. *Cancerland: A Medical Memoir*. New York: Thomas Dunne Books, 2018.

2. GOD'S PRESENCE ON DARK DAYS

Barton, Ruth Haley. *Sacred Rhythms: Arranging Our Lives for Spiritual Transformation*. Downers Grove, IL: InterVarsity Press, 2006.

Brother Lawrence with Harold Myra. *The Practice of the Presence of God*. Grand Rapids: Discovery House, 2017.

Foster, Richard. *Celebration of Discipline: The Path to Spiritual Growth*, spec. anniv. ed. New York: HarperOne, 2018.

Hayner, Steve, and Sharol Hayner. *Joy in the Journey: Finding Abundance in the Shadow of Death*. Downers Grove, IL: InterVarsity Press, 2015.

Nouwen, Henri. *Turn My Mourning into Dancing: Finding Hope in Hard Times*. Nashville: Thomas Nelson, 2001.

3. WHY ME?

Ford, Leighton. *Sandy: A Heart for God*. Downers Grove, IL: InterVarsity Press, 1985.

Groothuis, Douglas. *Walking Through Darkness: A Wife's Illness—A Philosopher's Lament*. Downers Grove, IL: InterVarsity Press, 2017.

Kapic, Kelly. *Embodied Hope: A Theological Meditation on Pain and Suffering*. Downers Grove, IL: InterVarsity Press, 2017.

Keller, Tim. *Walking with God Through Pain and Suffering*. New York: Dutton, 2013.

Sittser, Jerry. *A Grace Disguised: How the Soul Grows Through Loss*, exp. ed. Grand Rapids: Zondervan, 2004.

Tada, Joni Eareckson. *A Place of Healing: Wrestling with the Mysteries of Suffering, Pain, and God's Sovereignty*. Colorado Springs: Cook, 2010.

5. THE ILLUSION OF CONTROL

Heschel, Abraham. *The Sabbath*. New York: Farrar, Straus and Giroux, 1951.

Lucado, Max. *Anxious for Nothing: Finding Calm in a Chaotic World*. Nashville: Thomas Nelson, 2017.

Stott, John. *The Message of the Sermon on the Mount*. Bible Speaks Today. Downers Grove, IL: InterVarsity Press, 1978.

6. DEPENDING ON OTHERS

Bowler, Kate. *Everything Happens for a Reason and Other Lies I've Loved*. New York: Random House, 2018.

Farrow, John. *Damien the Leper*. New York: Image Books, 1954.

Mukherjee, Siddhartha. *The Emperor of All Maladies: A Biography of Cancer*. New York: Scribner, 2010.

7. IDENTITY

Stephenson, Robert Lewis. *The Strange Case of Dr. Jekyll and Mr. Hyde*. London: Dover Press, 1991.

Stott, John. *The Message of Ephesians*. Bible Speaks Today. Downers Grove, IL: InterVarsity Press, 1979.

Wilde, Oscar. *The Picture of Dorian Gray*. London: Dover Press, 2017.

8. SURVIVOR'S GROWTH

Feldman, David, and Lee Kravetz. *Supersurvivors: The Surprising Link Between Suffering and Success*. New York: HarperCollins, 2014.

Duckworth, Angela. *Grit: The Power of Passion and Perseverance*. New York: Scribner, 2016.

Rendon, Jim. *Upside: The New Science of Post-Traumatic Growth*. New York: Touchstone, 2015.

9. CLARITY OF PURPOSE

Card, Michael. *A Better Freedom: Finding Life as Slaves of Christ*. Downers Grove, IL: InterVarsity Press, 2009.

Ford, Leighton. *The Attentive Life: Discerning God's Presence in All Things*. Downers Grove, IL: InterVarsity Press, 2008.

Frankl, Viktor. *Man's Search for Meaning*. New York: Beacon Press, 2014.

10. REDEEMING TIME

Gawande, Atul. *Being Mortal: Medicine and What Matters at the End*. New York: Holt, 2014.

Kalanithi, Paul. *When Breath Becomes Air*. New York: Random House, 2016.

11. WONDER

Feinberg, Margaret. *Wonder Struck: Awaken to the Nearness of God*. Franklin, TN: Worthy Publishing, 2012.

Yaconelli, Michael. *Dangerous Wonder: The Adventure of Childlike Faith*. Colorado Springs: NavPress, 1998.

INDEX

ABOUT THE AUTHOR

A LEC HILL IS PRESIDENT EMERITUS of InterVarsity Christian Fellowship/USA. His primary focus is mentoring rising leaders. For fourteen years, he served as president before being diagnosed with cancer. He received a successful bone-marrow transplant from his brother Grant as donor. A year of quasi-isolation followed.

Prior to InterVarsity, Alec served as dean of the school of business and economics at Seattle Pacific University and professor of law and ethics. SPU has honored him both as Professor of the Year and Alumnus of the Year. He also served as regional director for World Relief.

Alec holds a law degree from the University of Washington as well as an MA in biblical literature and a BA in history from SPU. He has written widely in the fields of business ethics and the First Amendment. His book *Just Business: Christian Ethics for the Marketplace*, now in its third edition, has been translated into Chinese, Russian, Korean, and Indonesian.

He resides near Seattle with his wife, Mary, whom he has known since they were twelve and eleven years old, respectively. They have two daughters, Laura and Carolyn, both attorneys. He loves road trips, biographies, and the ill-fated Seattle Mariners. He serves as a visiting faculty member at Regent College (Canada) and as an adjunct instructor at SPU. He is also on the board of directors of Christianity Today.

ALSO BY THE AUTHOR

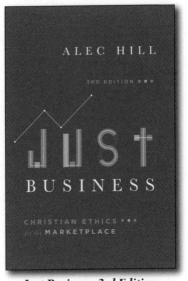

Just Business, 3rd Edition
978-0-8308-5198-0